Bradley Books

present

The 90-Day

Fitness Journal

Fat Gram
&
Calorie Counter
Including
Fast Foods

Plus...

**Low Fat, Low Calorie Recipes,
Exercise Tips, & More!**

Published in Minneapolis, Minnesota
by Bradley International Ltd.
4145 Parklawn Ave.
Suite 130
Edina, MN 55435

ISBN 0-9672367-0-3

Edited by Mary Ann Geiger and Martha Lundquist
Acknowledgements: Susan White, R.D., Nutrition Consultant
Cover illustration by Barry Lawrence, Edina, Minnesota

Dear Thin Within,

What if you were able to get in touch with someone who could guarantee that you'll lose weight? You can...that someone is *you!* Unfortunately, there's no magic pill; ultimately your success must come from within. You already know what it takes to lose weight—reduce calories and fat grams and increase your regular exercise. It's no easy task, but with accurate information, careful monitoring, and a desire to succeed, you'll soon be thinner and leading a healthier lifestyle.

Our goal is to give you every tool necessary to succeed at making permanent lifestyle changes. Our light-hearted quotes and hints are intended to inform, amuse, and encourage you while confronting what we know is a very serious issue.

As you complete your 90-day journal, you'll discover those factors that trigger over-eating—recognition is the first step toward a solution. You will see where your good intentions were sabotaged and you'll learn how to respond more appropriately to negative influences. This journal will help you to formulate a program that will keep the weight off and add years to your life.

You can do this! One day at a time, one step at a time, you're on your way!

Sincerely,

Brad Peterson

Brad Peterson,
President

Introduction

This book is unique because it offers you everything that you'll need to successfully lose weight—information, personal insight, and encouragement. It contains a 90-day section for monitoring your food choices, exercise, and other factors that influence your weight.

Everything you need is right here: a fat gram and calorie counter (including fast foods), an exercise chart, low-calorie recipes, hints for reducing fat in your cooking, and light-hearted quotes to encourage you on your road to improved fitness. By recording your food intake and exercise, you can determine where adjustments to your program are needed. The food value charts allow you to see where you can make healthier choices. You'll be surprised at how this charting will influence your future selections. Correlations between your emotions and eating habits will become obvious as you review your journal. Once you're alert to those factors that affect your weight, you'll be able to make positive behavioral changes. Soon you'll have a tailor-made program that works for *you!*

Table of Contents

On the Road to Fitness

Visualization

As you begin your journey to become more physically fit, take a moment to visualize how you'll look and feel after you lose weight. Imagine how great it will be to walk by a store window and admire your thinner reflection. The new-found self-assurance you'll acquire will put a spring in your step as you face each day with greater confidence.

On the following page, write down why you want to lose weight. Be specific—is it because you have to lower your blood pressure? Maybe you'd like to feel more attractive or perhaps have more years to enjoy with your children and grandchildren. Only you know your own personal reasons. Be very open and honest with yourself. Then write down how you imagine you'll look and feel after you get into shape. Your clothes will fit better, you'll be more physically active, and you'll have more confidence in all aspects of your life.

On those days when you need a little extra motivation and you feel more like flopping on the couch with a bag of chips than working out, look back at pages 10 and 11 in your journal. Those aspirations will give you the incentive to toss out the chips, get off the couch, and *just do it*—you're worth it!

Why I want to lose weight and become more physically fit:

_____

_____

_____

_____

_____

_____

_____

_____

_____

_____

_____

_____

_____

How I expect to look and feel once I'm thinner and healthier:

_____

_____

_____

_____

_____

_____

_____

_____

_____

_____

_____

_____

_____

_____

_____

_____

YAHOO!

Behavior Modification

Of all the people who are overweight, less than one percent of them can attribute their problem to a medical condition. Being overweight is often the result of learned behaviors. In addition to food choices, weight is affected by many emotional factors. Behavioral influences such as boredom, depression, and anger are just a few of the emotions that prompt one to turn to food for comfort. Eating makes stressful situations easier to tolerate. For years, perhaps for a lifetime, this pattern has become a learned behavior—one that has significantly contributed to weight problems.

The remedy is to learn *new* behaviors. It's much simpler to develop new habits than it is to lose old ones. With a commitment to establishing healthier behaviors, old habits will fade and be replaced by new ones. Eventually you'll notice a change in the way that you think about food.

The first step is to identify those environmental conditions that trigger your desire to eat. A food journal is an excellent way to do this. By writing down food items, portions, and the emotions that may have triggered an eating response, you will begin to develop an awareness of existing problem areas. Once you identify the pitfalls, you can take steps to correct or replace certain behaviors before reaching for food. Instead of eating, go for a walk, call a friend, take a relaxing soak in the tub, or do something else enjoyable.

Dining out is a good example of a situation that can present a challenge. You may feel that because you're paying for a meal, it's necessary to eat the whole thing...*wrong!* That's what "doggie bags" are for. Stop when you're no longer hungry and bring the rest home. Try sharing a meal with your dining companion. You might each order a cup of soup and then split an entree. Ask your server to bring sauces and dressings on the side and not to bring butter to the table.

Building a support system for yourself is important. It's so helpful to have even one or two other people encourage you by sharing recipes, joining you in physical activity, or cheering you on as you lose weight.

Try incorporating the following behavioral changes into your everyday lifestyle. Just a few small changes can make a big difference!

- Remove high calorie, high fat foods from your house.
- Eat slower; put your fork down between bites.
- Switch to skim milk instead of 2% or whole.
- Try not to sample food while you're cooking.
- Sit at the table for mealtime; don't eat standing up.
- Don't grocery shop when you're hungry.
- Make a grocery list before shopping and *stick to it!*
- Keep plenty of healthy foods in plain sight.
- Have desserts but make them 'lite.'
- A smaller plate will make your meal appear larger.
- Don't serve "family style." Keep extras in the kitchen.
- Cook without fat. Broil, bake, or poach instead.
- Sample different brands of low fat, low calorie foods.
- Be keenly aware of serving sizes.

You'll discover more behaviors that need to be changed as your personal pitfalls reveal themselves on the pages of your journal. Self-recognition is really the key. That's why it's so important to complete a journal page each day and then scrutinize your behavior. You can then prepare yourself to make better responses the next time those negative influences arise.

After you reach your desired weight, keep your journal handy. It can be helpful should you find destructive habits slipping back into your life. Reviewing your journal will help you to refocus on why it was important for you to become fit in the first place. Hopefully, that will motivate you to get back on track before things get too far out of hand.

Setting Realistic Goals

Your objective is to set achievable goals that won't harm your health but that still give you tangible and consistent weekly losses. Don't make the mistake of setting unrealistic goals that doom you to fail. It's more satisfying to *achieve* small goals than to fail at overly-ambitious ones. When you lose weight at a slower pace, you're more likely to keep that weight off. If you lose too much too fast, your body will try to fight the loss by slowing down your metabolism.

The more muscular you are, the more efficiently you burn calories. For example, if two people each weigh 200 pounds, the one with the greater percentage of muscle mass can consume more calories without gaining weight than the person who has a larger percentage of body fat. When you reduce your calories below what's believed to be a healthy level (about 1200-1500 calories per day depending upon your size and activity level), you may begin to burn not only stored body fat but muscle as well. That is exactly what you don't want to do.

When you set your calorie and fat gram allowances on the next few pages, keep in mind that in addition to setting an ultimate long-term goal, it's equally important to set several short-term goals. Attaining short-term goals will motivate you to stick with your program. You'll be continually adjusting your food choices until you've established nutritionally sound eating habits that you can live with forever.

Establishing Your Calorie Limits

First, the basics... a calorie is a unit of energy; 3,500 of these units (calories) equal one pound of stored body fat. To lose one pound of fat, you'll need to either reduce your caloric intake by 3,500 calories or burn that amount off through additional exercise (or better yet, a combination of the two).

Depending on one's level of activity, the average person requires about 12-15 calories per pound of body weight per day to maintain his or her current weight. For example, a 200-pound, reasonably active man probably consumes about 3,000 calories a day to maintain his weight (200 pounds x 15 calories per pound = 3,000 calories). If that 200-pound man reduces his calories to 2,500 a day, that 500 calorie reduction for seven days (500 x 7 = 3,500), will result in a one pound weight loss. If he eats 1,000 fewer calories per day, he will lose two pounds in seven days.

Most women lose an average of 1-2 pounds a week by consuming 1,200-1,500 calories a day. Most men lose 1-2 pounds a week by consuming 1,700-2,000 calories a day. A caloric intake below 1,200 calories is not recommended as these diets are often nutritionally inadequate.

If you're accustomed to consuming 3,000 calories a day and you cut back to 2,000 calories, you would lose two pounds per week. A healthy and practical goal would be 1½-2 pounds a week. If you're more than 50 pounds overweight, a 2½-3 pound per week weight loss would not be unreasonable. Set a realistic 90-day goal. This may not be your *ultimate* goal. It may be necessary to continue on until you reach your desired weight. Then set a two-week goal. Success in attaining short-term goals encourages you to continue on toward your ultimate goal.

In 90 days I'll lose_____pounds and I will weigh _____.

In 2 weeks I'll lose_____pounds.

My daily calorie allowance for the next two weeks is _____.

Note: Weigh yourself every two weeks, evaluate your progress, and set a new goal for the next two weeks. Resist the temptation to weigh yourself more frequently as water retention and other variables will affect your weight on a day-to-day basis. Fixating on *numbers* may cause you to focus less on the long-term objective.

Establishing Your Fat Gram Limits

A diet high in fat, especially saturated fat, causes elevated blood cholesterol levels in many people. High blood cholesterol increases the risk of heart disease, the nation's number one killer. A high-fat intake can also cause certain types of cancer, diabetes, and obesity. Reducing dietary fat is a good idea for everyone, especially those limiting calories to reduce weight. Fat has more than twice the calories of an equal weight of carbohydrate or protein. The fat in food provides many calories but few vitamins or minerals. Reducing fat intake almost always results in fewer calories.

On the average, Americans consume about 36% of their total calories as fat. Each gram of fat contains 9 calories. Many health agencies recommend limiting your fat intake to 30% or less of your total calories. Just how much fat is that? If you know about how many calories you usually eat each day, look at the following examples for the amounts of fat that equal 30% of calories.

• Sedentary women and young children would normally consume an average of 1,600 calories each day. Thirty percent of calories from fat equals 53 grams (1,600 x .30 = 480 ÷ 9 = 53.3, or 53 grams).

• Older children, teenage girls, active women, women who are pregnant or breast feeding, and many sedentary men consume about 2,200 calories each day. Thirty percent of calories from fat equals 73 grams (2,200 x .30 = 660 ÷ 9 = 73.3, or 73 grams).

• Teenage boys, active men, and some very active women consume about 2,800 calories a day. Thirty percent of calories from fat equals 93 fat grams (2,800 x .30 = 840 ÷ 9 = 93.3, or 93 fat grams).

Use the following formula to determine your maximum daily limit of fat grams based on the amount of calories you've allowed yourself each day.

_____ x .30 = _____ ÷ 9 = _____
Daily calorie   (%)   Calories   Fat gm.
allowance   per gram   per day

My daily fat gram allowance for the next two weeks is_____.

Note: The number you've determined as your fat gram allowance should be the maximum amount of fat that you consume per day. If you're able to reduce the percentage of fat in your diet to 25%, all the better.

Calorie Expenditure Chart

Activity	Calories per hr.
Aerobics (moderate)	400
Aerobics (intense)	890
Badminton	350
Bicycling (leisurely)	250
Bicycling (moderately)	400
Bowling	250
Canoeing	260
Gardening	240
Golf	250
Horseback riding	340
Housework	200
Ice skating	380
In-line skating	320
Jogging (5 mph)	550
Lawn mowing	240
Line dancing	280
Racquetball	560
Rowing (moderate)	400
Running (8 mph)	780
Skiing (cross-country)	900
Skiing (downhill)	560
Square dancing	380
Squash	620
Swimming (crawl)	800
Table tennis	350
Tennis (doubles)	320
Tennis (singles)	460
Volleyball	370
Walking (fast)	390
Walking (slow)	250
Water skiing	470

Exercise—Move It & Lose It!

Besides eating properly, another key ingredient to any long-term successful weight loss is exercise. Regular physical exercise increases your muscle strength and flexibility, strengthens your heart and lungs, burns calories, and just plain helps you feel better.

You should always check with your doctor before you start any exercise program, especially if you've been physically inactive. Your doctor can help you decide what activity is best for you or if there are any activities that you should avoid.

It's important to increase your percentage of muscle mass because pound for pound, muscle burns more calories than fat. This means that the more muscular your body is, the more efficiently it will burn calories. Increased muscle mass means that you can eat more calories without gaining weight!

A fitness program that combines aerobic exercises (like brisk walking or bicycling) with body strengthening exercises (such as weight training) yields optimal results. Aerobic-type exercises offer a cardiovascular workout and burn calories but do not build muscle mass. Body strengthening exercises build muscle mass. That's why it's important to incorporate both types of exercise into your workout program.

Increasing physical activity in even small ways such as taking the stairs instead of the elevator or by parking in a spot where you'll have to walk a greater distance will increase the number of calories you burn. It all adds up. Remember, whether you burn off 3,500 calories through exercise or reduce your caloric intake by 3,500 calories, you will lose one pound. And that, after all, *is* your objective.

You should make an effort to exercise at least three times a week. Your aerobic exercise should last no less than 20-30 minutes. Start out slowly if you've been inactive and gradually increase the length of your workout until you reach a minimum of 30 minutes. A program as simple as brisk walking every other day is a great start.

On page 20 you'll find an exercise chart that shows you about how many calories you'll burn when engaging in various types of exercise. These values represent averages. Your weight and muscle density will affect the rate at which you burn calories. A heavier, more muscular person will burn more calories during exercise, whereas a lighter, less muscular person will burn less calories performing the same exercises.

The key is consistency. That's why we've included a place for you to monitor your daily exercise. As you fill in your exercise data and see how many calories you've burned, you'll be motivated to stick with it. You'll find that you feel so much better when you exercise regularly that you'll want to make time for it each and every day.

Water—A Drink To Your Health

Last but not least, you will be monitoring the amount of water that you drink each day. Increasing your water intake helps to reduce fat deposits. Drinking at *least* eight 8-oz. glasses per day is very important for losing weight and keeping it off. As you lose weight, your body has to eliminate additional waste. The fat is metabolized and flushed out of your body by the water.

When water intake is insufficient, the liver is forced to do some of the kidney's work. This extra workload hinders the liver from properly metabolizing stored body fat into energy to fuel your body. This slows weight loss because you're burning less stored body fat.

Drink a couple of glasses of water one hour before you exercise, and another glass about 15 minutes before. If you're even slightly dehydrated you won't be able to perform at your peak. During competitive exercise your body can only absorb a pint or two of water per hour. When exercising moderately, it's not as essential, but still a good idea. An additional benefit to drinking lots of water is that it helps prevent your skin from sagging following weight loss.

A good time to drink a glass or two of water is about 20 minutes before having a meal. You'll tend to eat less because you'll feel the sensation of fullness more quickly. The heavier you are, the larger your metabolic load, therefore, the more water you'll need to drink. To keep you on track, each day in your journal contains eight boxes. Check off a box each time you drink an 8-oz. glass of water. These boxes will serve as a reminder to you to drink *all* eight glasses. **Note:** The water in coffee, tea, or other drinks does *not* count toward your eight glasses. Drink eight glasses of pure water in addition to other beverages.

Now that you're familiar with the various weight loss aspects that you'll be monitoring daily, it's time to start keeping your 90-day journal. Whenever possible, look up food values before eating rather than after so that you can see if you're spending your calories wisely. Be diligent about checking off the water boxes each time you finish a glass of water. Filling in the calories you burn each day through exercise will give you a sense of accomplishment. Most importantly, be candid when writing about emotional influences in the comments section of your journal. This way you can recognize where behavioral changes are needed. All of these components, working together, are what it takes to personalize a program for successful weight loss that will work for you. You're on your way to a healthier lifestyle!

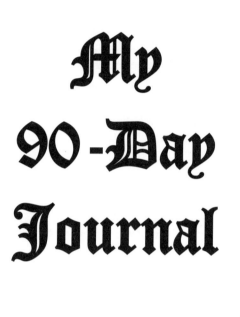

My
90-Day
Journal

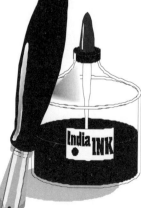

Day 28

Date __May 27__

Time & Place	Amt	Food	Cal.	Bal. 2000	Fat Gm.	Bal. 67
7 A.M. home	8 oz.	orange juice	110	1890	0	67
home	1 cup	Special K cereal	110	1780	0	67
	8 oz.	skim milk	90	1690	0	67
	4 slices	turkey bacon	80	1610	2	65
	1 cup	coffee	0	1610	0	65
	1 avg.	bagel	180	1430	2	63
	2 T.	cream cheese (lite)	70	1360	6	57
Noon McD.'s	1	McChicken sandwich	510	850	30	27
McD.'s	1	garden salad	50	800	2	25
	1 pkg.	vinaigrette (lite)	50	750	2	23
	1 cup	1% milk	100	650	3	20
	1	frozen yogurt sundae	210	440	1	19
5 P.M. Mom's	2 oz.	potato chips	300	140	18	1
Mom's	6 oz.	white wine	150	+10	0	1
	6 oz.	pork tenderloin (lean)	280	+290	8	+7
	1/2 cup	carrots	35	+325	0	+7
	1/2 cup	asparagus	20	+345	0	+7
	1 avg.	baked potato	150	+495	0	+7
	2 Tbsp.	sour cream (fat-free)	50	+545	0	+7
	1 cup	coffee	0	+545	0	+7
	2 Tbsp.	1/2 & 1/2	40	+585	3	+10

* This is a sample day for a 200-pound person with a weight loss goal of 2 pounds per week. Therefore, this person's daily allowances are 2,000 calories and 67 fat grams. Note: re-adjust calorie & fat gram allowances after each 10-pound weight loss.

Over by 585 calories and 10 fat gms. Get with it!!!

Ending Daily Balances +585 +10

26

Today's exercise   Duration

__*walked 3 miles (briskly)*__   __*45 minutes*__

_____   _____

Calories burned __*300*__

Check one box for each 8-oz. glass of water you drink

☑ ☑ ☑ ☑ ☑ ☑ ☐ ☐

It's Weigh Day!

SAMPLE

Starting weight __*210*__   **Today's weight** __*200*__

__*16*__ **pounds to lose until reaching 90-day goal.**

What's working? What's hindering? Revisions?

Drinking more water and adjusting to skim milk—Good!
Must look up food values ⟨before⟩ eating! A McGrilled
chicken sandwich would have saved me 26 fat grams &
250 calories! Snacking at Mom's after work is a prob-
lem—visit after dinner! Lots of pressure at work but
the walks help me to unwind. Sure beats eating!

My goal is to weigh __*196*__ **in two weeks.**

Date _____

Day 1

Time	Amt.	Food	Cal.	Bal.	Fat Gm.	Bal.

Ending Daily Balances

Today's exercise   Duration

_____   _____

_____   _____

Calories burned _____

Check one box for each 8-oz. glass of water you drink

☐   ☐   ☐   ☐   ☐   ☐   ☐   ☐

It's Weigh Day!

Starting weight _____   **Goal weight** _____

_____ **pounds to lose until reaching 90-day goal.**

What's working? What's hindering? Revisions?

_____

_____

_____

_____

_____

_____

My goal is to weigh _____ in two weeks.

Date _____

Day 2

Time	Amt.	Food	Cal.	Bal.	Fat Gm.	Bal.
		Ending Daily Balances				

Today's exercise   Duration

_____   _____

_____   _____

Calories burned _____

Check one box for each 8-oz. glass of water you drink

☐   ☐   ☐   ☐   ☐   ☐   ☐   ☐

Comments: _____

_____

_____

_____

_____

_____

_____

_____

_____

_____

_____

"The man who moves a mountain begins
by carrying small stones." —Chinese proverb

Date _____ **Day 3**

Time	Amt.	Food	Cal.	Bal.	Fat Gm.	Bal.
		Ending Daily Balances				

Today's exercise   Duration

_____   _____

_____   _____

Calories burned _____

Check one box for each 8-oz. glass of water you drink

☐ ☐ ☐ ☐ ☐ ☐ ☐ ☐

Comments: _____

_____

_____

_____

_____

_____

_____

_____

_____

"Never eat more than you can lift."
—Miss Piggy

Day 4

Time	Amt.	Food	Cal.	Bal.	Fat Gm.	Bal.
		Ending Daily Balances				

Today's exercise   Duration

_____   _____

_____   _____

Calories burned _____

Check one box for each 8-oz. glass of water you drink

☐ ☐ ☐ ☐ ☐ ☐ ☐ ☐

Comments: _____

_____

_____

_____

_____

_____

_____

_____

_____

_____

When preparing meat or poultry, cut off all
visible fat and remove the skin. Avoid breading
and coating mixes. Bake or broil; don't fry.

Date ——————— **Day 5**

Time	Amt.	Food	Cal.	Bal.	Fat Gm.	Bal.
		Ending Daily Balances				

Today's exercise   Duration

_____   _____

_____   _____

Calories burned _____

Check one box for each 8-oz. glass of water you drink

☐ ☐ ☐ ☐ ☐ ☐ ☐ ☐

Comments: _____

_____

_____

_____

_____

_____

_____

_____

_____

_____

Art Buchwald on liquid diets: "The powder is mixed
with water and tastes exactly like powder mixed with water."

Date _____ # Day 6

Time	Amt.	Food	Cal.	Bal.	Fat Gm.	Bal.
		Ending Daily Balances				

Today's exercise   Duration

_____   _____

_____   _____

Calories burned _____

Check one box for each 8-oz. glass of water you drink

☐ ☐ ☐ ☐ ☐ ☐ ☐ ☐

Comments: _____

_____

_____

_____

_____

_____

_____

_____

_____

_____

When eating out, ask your server to hold the
butter, mayo, or other sauces on your sandwich.
Ask for pretzels instead of chips or fries.

Date _____ **Day 7**

Time	Amt.	Food	Cal.	Bal.	Fat Gm.	Bal.
		Ending Daily Balances				

Today's exercise   Duration

_____   _____

_____   _____

Calories burned _____

Check one box for each 8-oz. glass of water you drink

☐ ☐ ☐ ☐ ☐ ☐ ☐ ☐

Comments: _____

_____

_____

_____

_____

_____

_____

_____

_____

_____

_____

Vary the types of exercises that you do; this will encompass
more muscles and prevent you from becoming bored.

Date ——————

Day 8

Time	Amt.	Food	Cal.	Bal.	Fat Gm.	Bal.
Ending Daily Balances						

Today's exercise   Duration

_____   _____

_____   _____

Calories burned _____

Check one box for each 8-oz. glass of water you drink

☐ ☐ ☐ ☐ ☐ ☐ ☐ ☐

Comments: _____

_____

_____

_____

_____

_____

_____

_____

_____

_____

You've hung in there for a full week! *Good for you!*
If you can do one week, you can do another. Keep
up the good work! You're on your way!

Day 9

Time	Amt.	Food	Cal.	Bal.	Fat Gm.	Bal.
		Ending Daily Balances				

Today's exercise   Duration

_____   _____

_____   _____

Calories burned _____

Check one box for each 8-oz. glass of water you drink

☐ ☐ ☐ ☐ ☐ ☐ ☐ ☐

Comments: _____

_____

_____

_____

_____

_____

_____

_____

_____

_____

Sampling food while cooking is a hidden pitfall.
Keep a dish of sliced fresh fruit or veggies to
nibble on or fix a juice spritzer or some tea.

Date ――――――――

Day 10

Time	Amt.	Food	Cal.	Bal.	Fat Gm.	Bal.
		Ending Daily Balances				

Today's exercise   Duration

_____   _____

_____   _____

Calories burned _____

Check one box for each 8-oz. glass of water you drink

☐ ☐ ☐ ☐ ☐ ☐ ☐ ☐

Comments: _____

_____

_____

_____

_____

_____

_____

_____

_____

_____

"Nature does her best to teach us. The
more we over-eat, the harder she makes it
for us to get close to the table." —Earl Wilson

Day 11

Time	Amt.	Food	Cal.	Bal.	Fat Gm.	Bal.
		Ending Daily Balances				

Today's exercise   Duration

_____   _____

_____   _____

Calories burned _____

Check one box for each 8-oz. glass of water you drink

☐ ☐ ☐ ☐ ☐ ☐ ☐ ☐

Comments: _____

_____

_____

_____

_____

_____

_____

_____

_____

_____

Have a designated eating area—ideally at the table.
Only eat when you're in that location. Serve your
food on a salad plate; it makes the plate look fuller.

Date _____

Day 12

Time	Amt.	Food	Cal.	Bal.	Fat Gm.	Bal.
		Ending Daily Balances				

Today's exercise   Duration

_____   _____

_____   _____

Calories burned _____

Check one box for each 8-oz. glass of water you drink

☐ ☐ ☐ ☐ ☐ ☐ ☐ ☐

Comments: _____

_____

_____

_____

_____

_____

_____

_____

_____

_____

Gradual transitions to low fat foods and then
to non-fat foods can be an effective approach if
you're having difficulty making eating changes.

Date _____

Day 13

Time	Amt.	Food	Cal.	Bal.	Fat Gm.	Bal.
		Ending Daily Balances				

Today's exercise   Duration

_____   _____

_____   _____

Calories burned _____

Check one box for each 8-oz. glass of water you drink

☐ ☐ ☐ ☐ ☐ ☐ ☐ ☐

Comments: _____

_____

_____

_____

_____

_____

_____

_____

_____

_____

_____

The weight reducer is one who has learned that what's
on the table eventually becomes what's on the chair.

Date _____ # Day 14

Time	Amt.	Food	Cal.	Bal.	Fat Gm.	Bal.
		Ending Daily Balances				

Today's exercise   Duration

_____   _____

_____   _____

Calories burned _____

Check one box for each 8-oz. glass of water you drink

☐ ☐ ☐ ☐ ☐ ☐ ☐ ☐

Comments: _____

_____

_____

_____

_____

_____

_____

_____

_____

_____

_____

"A good reducing exercise consists of placing both hands
against the table edge and pushing back." —Robert Quillen

Date _____   # Day 15

Time	Amt.	Food	Cal.	Bal.	Fat Gm.	Bal.
		Ending Daily Balances				

Today's exercise   Duration

_____   _____

_____   _____

Calories burned _____

Check one box for each 8-oz. glass of water you drink

☐   ☐   ☐   ☐   ☐   ☐   ☐   ☐

It's Weigh Day!

Starting weight _____ **Today's weight** _____
_____ **pounds to lose until reaching 90-day goal.**

What's working? What's hindering? Revisions?

_____

_____

_____

_____

_____

_____

My goal is to weigh _____ in two weeks.

Date _____   # Day 16

Time	Amt.	Food	Cal.	Bal.	Fat Gm.	Bal.
		Ending Daily Balances				

Today's exercise   Duration

_____   _____

_____   _____

Calories burned _____

Check one box for each 8-oz. glass of water you drink

☐   ☐   ☐   ☐   ☐   ☐   ☐   ☐

Comments: _____

_____

_____

_____

_____

_____

_____

_____

_____

_____

Make a grocery list before shopping and *stick to it!*
Never shop when you're hungry or you're likely to
be tempted by enticing displays or packaging.

Date ——————— **Day 17**

Time	Amt.	Food	Cal.	Bal.	Fat Gm.	Bal.
		Ending Daily Balances				

Today's exercise   Duration

_____   _____

_____   _____

Calories burned _____

Check one box for each 8-oz. glass of water you drink

☐ ☐ ☐ ☐ ☐ ☐ ☐ ☐

Comments: _____

_____

_____

_____

_____

_____

_____

_____

_____

_____

_____

"Desperation is a fellow shaving before
stepping on the scale." —Anonymous

Date _____   **Day 18**

Time	Amt.	Food	Cal.	Bal.	Fat Gm.	Bal.
		Ending Daily Balances				

Today's exercise   Duration

_____   _____

_____   _____

Calories burned _____

Check one box for each 8-oz. glass of water you drink

☐   ☐   ☐   ☐   ☐   ☐   ☐   ☐

Comments: _____

_____

_____

_____

_____

_____

_____

_____

_____

_____

Steam vegetables to help retain their vitamins. Try flavoring them with lemon or lime juice instead of butter. Potatoes are healthy. Bake or boil them; just don't cook them in oil or fat.

Date ———————

Day 19

Time	Amt.	Food	Cal.	Bal.	Fat Gm.	Bal.
		Ending Daily Balances				

Today's exercise   Duration

_____   _____

_____   _____

           Calories burned _____

Check one box for each 8-oz. glass of water you drink

☐   ☐   ☐   ☐   ☐   ☐   ☐   ☐

Comments: _____

_____

_____

_____

_____

_____

_____

_____

_____

_____

_____

"At least half of the exercise I get every day comes
from jumping to conclusions." —Bruce Dexter

Date ———————

Day 20

Time	Amt.	Food	Cal.	Bal.	Fat Gm.	Bal.
		Ending Daily Balances				

Today's exercise   Duration

_____   _____

_____   _____

Calories burned _____

Check one box for each 8-oz. glass of water you drink

☐ ☐ ☐ ☐ ☐ ☐ ☐ ☐

Comments: _____

_____

_____

_____

_____

_____

_____

_____

_____

_____

If you lose weight quickly, you're likely to gain it back
rapidly. Fad diets do not contain the vitamins and minerals
necessary for good health. Slow and steady works best.

Date —————— **Day 21**

Time	Amt.	Food	Cal.	Bal.	Fat Gm.	Bal.
		Ending Daily Balances				

Today's exercise   Duration

_____   _____

_____   _____

Calories burned _____

Check one box for each 8-oz. glass of water you drink

☐   ☐   ☐   ☐   ☐   ☐   ☐   ☐

Comments: _____

_____

_____

_____

_____

_____

_____

_____

_____

_____

_____

"I don't work out. If God wanted us to bend over,
He'd put diamonds on the floor." —Joan Rivers

Date _____ **Day 22**

Time	Amt.	Food	Cal.	Bal.	Fat Gm.	Bal.
		Ending Daily Balances				

Today's exercise   Duration

_____   _____

_____   _____

Calories burned _____

Check one box for each 8-oz. glass of water you drink

☐ ☐ ☐ ☐ ☐ ☐ ☐ ☐

Comments: _____

_____

_____

_____

_____

_____

_____

_____

_____

_____

Three weeks and you're still going strong!
Great job! Small changes are beginning to
make big differences. You're on the right road!

Day 23

Time	Amt.	Food	Cal.	Bal.	Fat Gm.	Bal.
		Ending Daily Balances				

Today's exercise   Duration

_____   _____

_____   _____

Calories burned _____

Check one box for each 8-oz. glass of water you drink

☐ ☐ ☐ ☐ ☐ ☐ ☐ ☐

Comments: _____

_____

_____

_____

_____

_____

_____

_____

_____

_____

Serve plenty of chilled veggies, fruit, and juices to
your children and grandchildren. This will teach them
to enjoy healthy food choices for a lifetime of fitness.

Date _____ **Day 24**

Time	Amt.	Food	Cal.	Bal.	Fat Gm.	Bal.
		Ending Daily Balances				

Today's exercise   Duration

_____   _____

_____   _____

Calories burned _____

Check one box for each 8-oz. glass of water you drink

☐ ☐ ☐ ☐ ☐ ☐ ☐ ☐

Comments: _____

_____

_____

_____

_____

_____

_____

_____

_____

_____

Ideal weight: the weight listed
on a person's driver's license.

Date ——————— **Day 25**

Time	Amt.	Food	Cal.	Bal.	Fat Gm.	Bal.
		Ending Daily Balances				

Today's exercise   Duration

_____   _____

_____   _____

Calories burned _____

Check one box for each 8-oz. glass of water you drink

☐ ☐ ☐ ☐ ☐ ☐ ☐ ☐

Comments: _____

_____

_____

_____

_____

_____

_____

_____

_____

_____

Enjoy potato skins? No need to give them up! Coat a cookie
sheet with non-fat spray; sprinkle the potato skins or thin
slices with garlic salt, pepper, and paprika. Broil until crisp.

Date _____ # Day 26

Time	Amt.	Food	Cal.	Bal.	Fat Gm.	Bal.
		Ending Daily Balances				

Today's exercise   Duration

_____   _____

_____   _____

Calories burned _____

Check one box for each 8-oz. glass of water you drink

☐ ☐ ☐ ☐ ☐ ☐ ☐ ☐

Comments: _____

_____

_____

_____

_____

_____

_____

_____

_____

_____

_____

Strawberries dipped in powdered sugar
make a simple, elegant, and fat-free dessert.

Date ——————

Day 27

Time	Amt.	Food	Cal.	Bal.	Fat Gm.	Bal.
		Ending Daily Balances				

Today's exercise   Duration

_____   _____

_____   _____

Calories burned _____

Check one box for each 8-oz. glass of water you drink

☐   ☐   ☐   ☐   ☐   ☐   ☐   ☐

Comments: _____

_____

_____

_____

_____

_____

_____

_____

_____

_____

"If I'd known how long I was going to live,
I'd have taken better care of myself."
—Adolph Zukor at age 99

Date _____   **Day 28**

Time	Amt.	Food	Cal.	Bal.	Fat Gm.	Bal.
		Ending Daily Balances				

Today's exercise   Duration

_____   _____

_____   _____

Calories burned _____

Check one box for each 8-oz. glass of water you drink

☐   ☐   ☐   ☐   ☐   ☐   ☐   ☐

Comments: _____

_____

_____

_____

_____

_____

_____

_____

_____

_____

Add extra fruit to your meals. Try adding grapes
or mandarin oranges to tuna or chicken salads.

Day 29

Date _____

Time	Amt.	Food	Cal.	Bal.	Fat Gm.	Bal.
		Ending Daily Balances				

Today's exercise   Duration

_____   _____

_____   _____

Calories burned _____

Check one box for each 8-oz. glass of water you drink

☐   ☐   ☐   ☐   ☐   ☐   ☐   ☐

It's Weigh Day!

Starting weight _____ **Today's weight** _____
_____ **pounds to lose until reaching 90-day goal.**

What's working? What's hindering? Revisions?

_____

_____

_____

_____

_____

_____

My goal is to weigh _____ **in two weeks.**

Date _____ **Day 30**

Time	Amt.	Food	Cal.	Bal.	Fat Gm.	Bal.
		Ending Daily Balances				

Today's exercise   Duration

_____   _____

_____   _____

Calories burned _____

Check one box for each 8-oz. glass of water you drink

☐   ☐   ☐   ☐   ☐   ☐   ☐   ☐

Comments: _____

_____

_____

_____

_____

_____

_____

_____

_____

_____

"Whether you think you can or think
you can't—you're right." —Henry Ford

Date ―――――――

Day 31

Time	Amt.	Food	Cal.	Bal.	Fat Gm.	Bal.
		Ending Daily Balances				

Today's exercise   Duration

_____   _____

_____   _____

Calories burned _____

Check one box for each 8-oz. glass of water you drink

☐ ☐ ☐ ☐ ☐ ☐ ☐ ☐

Comments: _____

_____

_____

_____

_____

_____

_____

_____

_____

_____

Add thin-sliced cucumber, tomato, lettuce,
or sprouts to your sandwiches. It makes
them more filling and nutritious.

Day 32

Time	Amt.	Food	Cal.	Bal.	Fat Gm.	Bal.

Ending Daily Balances

Today's exercise   Duration

_____   _____

_____   _____

            Calories burned _____

Check one box for each 8-oz. glass of water you drink

☐   ☐   ☐   ☐   ☐   ☐   ☐   ☐

Comments: _____

_____

_____

_____

_____

_____

_____

_____

_____

_____

"From the day on which she weighs 140, the chief
excitement in a woman's life consists of spotting
women who are fatter than she is." —Helen Rowland

Date _____ **Day 33**

Time	Amt.	Food	Cal.	Bal.	Fat Gm.	Bal.
		Ending Daily Balances				

Today's exercise   Duration

_____   _____

_____   _____

Calories burned _____

Check one box for each 8-oz. glass of water you drink

☐ ☐ ☐ ☐ ☐ ☐ ☐ ☐

Comments: _____

_____

_____

_____

_____

_____

_____

_____

_____

_____

_____

Just as an architect needs a blueprint, you must
have an exercise plan and be sure to stick with it.

Date _____ # Day 34

Time	Amt.	Food	Cal.	Bal.	Fat Gm.	Bal.
		Ending Daily Balances				

Today's exercise   Duration

_____   _____

_____   _____

Calories burned _____

Check one box for each 8-oz. glass of water you drink

☐ ☐ ☐ ☐ ☐ ☐ ☐ ☐

Comments: _____

_____

_____

_____

_____

_____

_____

_____

_____

_____

Weight: what a man always
loses when his wife is on a diet.

Date _____

Day 35

Time	Amt.	Food	Cal.	Bal.	Fat Gm.	Bal.
Ending Daily Balances						

Today's exercise   Duration

_____   _____

_____   _____

Calories burned _____

Check one box for each 8-oz. glass of water you drink

☐ ☐ ☐ ☐ ☐ ☐ ☐ ☐

Comments: _____

_____

_____

_____

_____

_____

_____

_____

_____

_____

_____

"When it comes to eating, you can sometimes help
yourself more by helping yourself less." —Richard Amore

Date _____

Day 36

Time	Amt.	Food	Cal.	Bal.	Fat Gm.	Bal.
		Ending Daily Balances				

Today's exercise   Duration

_____   _____

_____   _____

Calories burned _____

Check one box for each 8-oz. glass of water you drink

☐ ☐ ☐ ☐ ☐ ☐ ☐ ☐

Comments: _____

_____

_____

_____

_____

_____

_____

_____

_____

_____

Five weeks—that's great! You can be proud of yourself. Don't
worry if your weight loss plateaus occasionally. That's not
uncommon. Stick with your new habits and you'll lose weight.

Date _____   **Day 37**

Time	Amt.	Food	Cal.	Bal.	Fat Gm.	Bal.
		Ending Daily Balances				

Today's exercise   Duration

_____   _____

_____   _____

Calories burned _____

Check one box for each 8-oz. glass of water you drink

☐ ☐ ☐ ☐ ☐ ☐ ☐ ☐

Comments: _____

_____

_____

_____

_____

_____

_____

_____

_____

_____

_____

When recipes call for eggs, use egg substitutes
or separate the eggs using just the egg whites.

Date —————— # Day 38

Time	Amt.	Food	Cal.	Bal.	Fat Gm.	Bal.
		Ending Daily Balances				

Today's exercise   Duration

_____   _____

_____   _____

Calories burned _____

Check one box for each 8-oz. glass of water you drink

☐ ☐ ☐ ☐ ☐ ☐ ☐ ☐

Comments: _____

_____

_____

_____

_____

_____

_____

_____

_____

_____

"I eat merely to put food out of my mind."
—N.F. Simpson

Date ———————

Day 39

Time	Amt.	Food	Cal.	Bal.	Fat Gm.	Bal.
Ending Daily Balances						

Today's exercise   Duration

_____   _____

_____   _____

Calories burned _____

Check one box for each 8-oz. glass of water you drink

☐ ☐ ☐ ☐ ☐ ☐ ☐ ☐

Comments: _____

_____

_____

_____

_____

_____

_____

_____

_____

_____

Substitute chicken broth, vegetable broth, or
white wine for some of the olive oil called for
in pesto and other oil-based sauces for pasta.

Date ——————

Day 40

Time	Amt.	Food	Cal.	Bal.	Fat Gm.	Bal.
		Ending Daily Balances				

Today's exercise   Duration

_____   _____

_____   _____

Calories burned _____

Check one box for each 8-oz. glass of water you drink

☐ ☐ ☐ ☐ ☐ ☐ ☐ ☐

Comments: _____

_____

_____

_____

_____

_____

_____

_____

_____

_____

"God must have loved calories because
He made so many of them!" —Anonymous

Date ———————

Day 41

Time	Amt.	Food	Cal.	Bal.	Fat Gm.	Bal.
		Ending Daily Balances				

Today's exercise   Duration

_____   _____

_____   _____

Calories burned _____

Check one box for each 8-oz. glass of water you drink

☐ ☐ ☐ ☐ ☐ ☐ ☐ ☐

Comments: _____

_____

_____

_____

_____

_____

_____

_____

_____

_____

Reduce cheese in your recipes as much as
possible. Cut amounts called for in half as
each ounce contains about 10 grams of fat.

Date _____   # Day 42

Time	Amt.	Food	Cal.	Bal.	Fat Gm.	Bal.
		Ending Daily Balances				

Today's exercise   Duration

_____   _____

_____   _____

Calories burned _____

Check one box for each 8-oz. glass of water you drink

☐ ☐ ☐ ☐ ☐ ☐ ☐ ☐

Comments: _____

_____

_____

_____

_____

_____

_____

_____

_____

_____

_____

The longer you cook fatty meats, the less fat is left.
When reducing, order your meat medium to well-done.

Date —————— **Day 43**

Time	Amt.	Food	Cal.	Bal.	Fat Gm.	Bal.
		Ending Daily Balances				

Today's exercise   Duration

_____   _____

_____   _____

Calories burned _____

Check one box for each 8-oz. glass of water you drink

☐   ☐   ☐   ☐   ☐   ☐   ☐   ☐

It's Weigh Day!

Starting weight _____ **Today's weight** _____
_____ **pounds to lose until reaching 90-day goal.**

What's working? What's hindering? Revisions?

_____

_____

_____

_____

_____

_____

My goal is to weigh _____ **in two weeks.**

Day 44

Time	Amt.	Food	Cal.	Bal.	Fat Gm.	Bal.
		Ending Daily Balances				

Today's exercise

Duration

_____

_____

_____

_____

Calories burned _____

Check one box for each 8-oz. glass of water you drink

☐ ☐ ☐ ☐ ☐ ☐ ☐ ☐

Comments: _____

_____

_____

_____

_____

_____

_____

_____

_____

_____

There's a new invention on the market for people
on diets—an ice cream bar with lettuce on the inside.

Date _____ # Day 45

Time	Amt.	Food	Cal.	Bal.	Fat Gm.	Bal.
		Ending Daily Balances				

Today's exercise   Duration

_____   _____

_____   _____

Calories burned _____

Check one box for each 8-oz. glass of water you drink

☐　☐　☐　☐　☐　☐　☐　☐

Comments: _____

_____

_____

_____

_____

_____

_____

_____

_____

_____

For an easy apple cobbler, mix apple slices, raisins,
and brown sugar. Microwave. Add skim milk.

Date _____ # Day 46

Time	Amt.	Food	Cal.	Bal.	Fat Gm.	Bal.
		Ending Daily Balances				

Today's exercise   Duration

_____   _____

_____   _____

Calories burned _____

Check one box for each 8-oz. glass of water you drink

☐ ☐ ☐ ☐ ☐ ☐ ☐ ☐

Comments: _____

_____

_____

_____

_____

_____

_____

_____

_____

_____

_____

When eating out, ask your server to bring your salad dressing
on the side. Dip your fork prongs into the dressing and then
the salad. You'll still enjoy the taste while eating less dressing.

Date _____ **Day 47**

Time	Amt.	Food	Cal.	Bal.	Fat Gm.	Bal.
		Ending Daily Balances				

Today's exercise   Duration

_____   _____

_____   _____

Calories burned _____

Check one box for each 8-oz. glass of water you drink

☐ ☐ ☐ ☐ ☐ ☐ ☐ ☐

Comments: _____

_____

_____

_____

_____

_____

_____

_____

_____

_____

Another great reducing exercise: shake your head
vigorously from side to side when offered a second helping.

Day 48

Date _____

Time	Amt.	Food	Cal.	Bal.	Fat Gm.	Bal.
			Ending Daily Balances			

Today's exercise   Duration

_____   _____

_____   _____

Calories burned _____

Check one box for each 8-oz. glass of water you drink

☐ ☐ ☐ ☐ ☐ ☐ ☐ ☐

Comments: _____

_____

_____

_____

_____

_____

_____

_____

_____

_____

Reduce fat in a meat loaf by eliminating the loaf pan.
Place rounded loaves on a broiling pan and bake. Fat drips
through to the lower pan and doesn't stay in the loaf.

Day 49

Date _____

Time	Amt.	Food	Cal.	Bal.	Fat Gm.	Bal.
		Ending Daily Balances				

Today's exercise   Duration

_____   _____

_____   _____

Calories burned _____

Check one box for each 8-oz. glass of water you drink

☐   ☐   ☐   ☐   ☐   ☐   ☐   ☐

Comments: _____

_____

_____

_____

_____

_____

_____

_____

_____

_____

"I don't know why I even waste time eating this food. I should
just apply it directly to my hips." —Rhoda Morgenstern

Date ───────── **Day 50**

Time	Amt.	Food	Cal.	Bal.	Fat Gm.	Bal.
		Ending Daily Balances				

Today's exercise   Duration

_____   _____

_____   _____

Calories burned _____

Check one box for each 8-oz. glass of water you drink

☐ ☐ ☐ ☐ ☐ ☐ ☐ ☐

Comments: _____

_____

_____

_____

_____

_____

_____

_____

_____

_____

It's actually been seven weeks! You're more than half way
through your 90-day plan. You should be very proud of yourself!

Date ——————— **Day 51**

Time	Amt.	Food	Cal.	Bal.	Fat Gm.	Bal.
		Ending Daily Balances				

Today's exercise

Duration

_____

_____

_____

_____

Calories burned _____

Check one box for each 8-oz. glass of water you drink

☐ ☐ ☐ ☐ ☐ ☐ ☐ ☐

Comments: _____

_____

_____

_____

_____

_____

_____

_____

_____

_____

_____

"As a child, my family's menu consisted of two
choices—take it or leave it." —Buddy Hackett

Date ——————————

Day 52

Time	Amt.	Food	Cal.	Bal.	Fat Gm.	Bal.
		Ending Daily Balances				

Today's exercise   Duration

_____   _____

_____   _____

Calories burned _____

Check one box for each 8-oz. glass of water you drink

☐ ☐ ☐ ☐ ☐ ☐ ☐ ☐

Comments: _____

_____

_____

_____

_____

_____

_____

_____

_____

_____

Eat according to your body signals. Getting overly-hungry
just sets you up to over-eat when you finally have a meal.

Date _____

Day 53

Time	Amt.	Food	Cal.	Bal.	Fat Gm.	Bal.
		Ending Daily Balances				

Today's exercise   Duration

_____   _____

_____   _____

Calories burned _____

Check one box for each 8-oz. glass of water you drink

☐ ☐ ☐ ☐ ☐ ☐ ☐ ☐

Comments: _____

_____

_____

_____

_____

_____

_____

_____

_____

_____

"Life itself is the proper binge."
—Julia Child

Date _____ **Day 54**

Time	Amt.	Food	Cal.	Bal.	Fat Gm.	Bal.
		Ending Daily Balances				

Today's exercise   Duration

_____   _____

_____   _____

            Calories burned _____

Check one box for each 8-oz. glass of water you drink

☐ ☐ ☐ ☐ ☐ ☐ ☐ ☐

Comments: _____

_____

_____

_____

_____

_____

_____

_____

_____

_____

"Oh Lord, if you can't make me look thin,
then please make my friends look fat."
—Erma Bombeck

Date _____   # Day 55

Time	Amt.	Food	Cal.	Bal.	Fat Gm.	Bal.
		Ending Daily Balances				

Today's exercise   Duration

_____   _____

_____   _____

Calories burned _____

Check one box for each 8-oz. glass of water you drink

☐ ☐ ☐ ☐ ☐ ☐ ☐ ☐

Comments: _____

_____

_____

_____

_____

_____

_____

_____

_____

_____

For a tasty baked potato without fatty
topping, try salsa. It's surprisingly good!

Date _____

Day 56

Time	Amt.	Food	Cal.	Bal.	Fat Gm.	Bal.
		Ending Daily Balances				

Today's exercise   Duration

_____   _____

_____   _____

Calories burned _____

Check one box for each 8-oz. glass of water you drink

☐ ☐ ☐ ☐ ☐ ☐ ☐ ☐

Comments: _____

_____

_____

_____

_____

_____

_____

_____

_____

_____

"Thin people are beautiful, but fat
people are adorable." —Jackie Gleason

Date ―――――――― **Day 57**

Time	Amt.	Food	Cal.	Bal.	Fat Gm.	Bal.
		Ending Daily Balances				

Today's exercise   Duration

_____   _____

_____   _____

Calories burned _____

Check one box for each 8-oz. glass of water you drink

☐   ☐   ☐   ☐   ☐   ☐   ☐   ☐

It's Weigh Day!

Starting weight _____ **Today's weight** _____

_____ **pounds to lose until reaching 90-day goal.**

What's working? What's hindering? Revisions?

_____

_____

_____

_____

_____

_____

My goal is to weigh _____ **in two weeks.**

Day 58

Time	Amt.	Food	Cal.	Bal.	Fat Gm.	Bal.
		Ending Daily Balances				

Today's exercise   Duration

_____   _____

_____   _____

                Calories burned _____

Check one box for each 8-oz. glass of water you drink

☐   ☐   ☐   ☐   ☐   ☐   ☐   ☐

Comments: _____

_____

_____

_____

_____

_____

_____

_____

_____

_____

Expand your horizons—make a point of
trying a new fruit or vegetable each week.

Date _____   # Day 59

Time	Amt.	Food	Cal.	Bal.	Fat Gm.	Bal.
		Ending Daily Balances				

Today's exercise   Duration

_____   _____

_____   _____

Calories burned _____

Check one box for each 8-oz. glass of water you drink

☐ ☐ ☐ ☐ ☐ ☐ ☐ ☐

Comments: _____

_____

_____

_____

_____

_____

_____

_____

_____

_____

Whenever possible keep fruits, vegetables, or bagels in a small cooler and take them with you each day. When healthy foods are available, you'll be less likely to buy junk food.

Date —————   # Day 60

Time	Amt.	Food	Cal.	Bal.	Fat Gm.	Bal.
		Ending Daily Balances				

Today's exercise   Duration

_____   _____

_____   _____

Calories burned _____

Check one box for each 8-oz. glass of water you drink

☐ ☐ ☐ ☐ ☐ ☐ ☐ ☐

Comments: _____

_____

_____

_____

_____

_____

_____

_____

_____

_____

"Remember, *never* exercise between meals!"
—Miss Piggy

Date ――――――― **Day 61**

Time	Amt.	Food	Cal.	Bal.	Fat Gm.	Bal.
		Ending Daily Balances				

Today's exercise   Duration

_____   _____

_____   _____

Calories burned _____

Check one box for each 8-oz. glass of water you drink

☐ ☐ ☐ ☐ ☐ ☐ ☐ ☐

Comments: _____

_____

_____

_____

_____

_____

_____

_____

_____

_____

One good thing about being in rotten physical
shape—at least you don't have to exercise to keep it up.

Date _____

Day 62

Time	Amt.	Food	Cal.	Bal.	Fat Gm.	Bal.
		Ending Daily Balances				

Today's exercise   Duration

_____   _____

_____   _____

Calories burned _____

Check one box for each 8-oz. glass of water you drink

☐ ☐ ☐ ☐ ☐ ☐ ☐ ☐

Comments: _____

_____

_____

_____

_____

_____

_____

_____

_____

_____

_____

Obstacles are things people see when
they take their eyes off a goal.

Date —————— **Day 63**

Time	Amt.	Food	Cal.	Bal.	Fat Gm.	Bal.
		Ending Daily Balances				

Today's exercise   Duration

_____   _____

_____   _____

Calories burned _____

Check one box for each 8-oz. glass of water you drink

☐   ☐   ☐   ☐   ☐   ☐   ☐   ☐

Comments: _____

_____

_____

_____

_____

_____

_____

_____

_____

_____

Walking a mile will burn as many calories as jogging a
mile and will only put a third of the pressure on your joints.

Date _____ **Day 64**

Time	Amt.	Food	Cal.	Bal.	Fat Gm.	Bal.
		Ending Daily Balances				

Today's exercise   Duration

_____   _____

_____   _____

Calories burned   _____

Check one box for each 8-oz. glass of water you drink

☐ ☐ ☐ ☐ ☐ ☐ ☐ ☐

Comments: _____

_____

_____

_____

_____

_____

_____

_____

_____

_____

It's been nine weeks! What perseverance! Why not
have a massage or a facial today—you deserve it!

Date _____ # Day 65

Time	Amt.	Food	Cal.	Bal.	Fat Gm.	Bal.
		Ending Daily Balances				

Today's exercise   Duration

_____   _____

_____   _____

Calories burned _____

Check one box for each 8-oz. glass of water you drink

☐ ☐ ☐ ☐ ☐ ☐ ☐ ☐

Comments: _____

_____

_____

_____

_____

_____

_____

_____

_____

_____

_____

"I'm on a seafood diet. Every time
I see food, I eat it." —Anonymous

Date _____

Day 66

Time	Amt.	Food	Cal.	Bal.	Fat Gm.	Bal.
		Ending Daily Balances				

Today's exercise   Duration

_____   _____

_____   _____

Calories burned _____

Check one box for each 8-oz. glass of water you drink

☐ ☐ ☐ ☐ ☐ ☐ ☐ ☐

Comments: _____

_____

_____

_____

_____

_____

_____

_____

_____

_____

"The trouble with jogging is by the time you realize
you're not in shape for it, it's too far to walk back."
—Franklin P. Jones

Date _____ **Day 67**

Time	Amt.	Food	Cal.	Bal.	Fat Gm.	Bal.
		Ending Daily Balances				

Today's exercise   Duration

_____   _____

_____   _____

Calories burned _____

Check one box for each 8-oz. glass of water you drink

☐ ☐ ☐ ☐ ☐ ☐ ☐ ☐

Comments: _____

_____

_____

_____

_____

_____

_____

_____

_____

_____

Use lettuce leaves instead of a tortilla for a tasty, low calorie burrito. Fill it with meat, low fat cheese, veggies, and salsa.

Date _____   **Day 68**

Time	Amt.	Food	Cal.	Bal.	Fat Gm.	Bal.
		Ending Daily Balances				

Today's exercise   Duration

_____   _____

_____   _____

Calories burned _____

Check one box for each 8-oz. glass of water you drink

☐   ☐   ☐   ☐   ☐   ☐   ☐   ☐

Comments: _____

_____

_____

_____

_____

_____

_____

_____

_____

_____

_____

Sandwich spread—what you
get from eating between meals.

Date _____

Day 69

Time	Amt.	Food	Cal.	Bal.	Fat Gm.	Bal.
		Ending Daily Balances				

Today's exercise   Duration

_____   _____

_____   _____

Calories burned _____

Check one box for each 8-oz. glass of water you drink

☐ ☐ ☐ ☐ ☐ ☐ ☐ ☐

Comments: _____

_____

_____

_____

_____

_____

_____

_____

_____

_____

"Everyone loves a fat man—until
he sits down on a bus." —Anonymous

Date ———————

Day 70

Time	Amt.	Food	Cal.	Bal.	Fat Gm.	Bal.
		Ending Daily Balances				

Today's exercise   Duration

_____   _____

_____   _____

Calories burned _____

Check one box for each 8-oz. glass of water you drink

☐   ☐   ☐   ☐   ☐   ☐   ☐   ☐

Comments: _____

_____

_____

_____

_____

_____

_____

_____

_____

_____

_____

"You know you've lost too much weight when panhandlers
give you money and tell you to get a hot meal." —Anonymous

Date _____ **Day 71**

Time	Amt.	Food	Cal.	Bal.	Fat Gm.	Bal.
		Ending Daily Balances				

Today's exercise   Duration

_____   _____

_____   _____

Calories burned _____

Check one box for each 8-oz. glass of water you drink

☐ ☐ ☐ ☐ ☐ ☐ ☐ ☐

It's Weigh Day!

Starting weight _____ **Today's weight** _____
_____ **pounds to lose until reaching 90-day goal.**

What's working? What's hindering? Revisions?

_____

_____

_____

_____

_____

_____

My goal is to weigh _____ **in two weeks.**

Date _____

Day 72

Time	Amt.	Food	Cal.	Bal.	Fat Gm.	Bal.
		Ending Daily Balances				

Today's exercise   Duration

_____   _____

_____   _____

Calories burned _____

Check one box for each 8-oz. glass of water you drink

☐ ☐ ☐ ☐ ☐ ☐ ☐ ☐

Comments: _____

_____

_____

_____

_____

_____

_____

_____

_____

_____

_____

Keep higher calorie foods in the back of the
refrigerator or on the top cupboard shelf. Store
healthier items where they're more accessible.

Date _____ # Day 73

Time	Amt.	Food	Cal.	Bal.	Fat Gm.	Bal.
		Ending Daily Balances				

Today's exercise   Duration

_____   _____

_____   _____

Calories burned _____

Check one box for each 8-oz. glass of water you drink

☐ ☐ ☐ ☐ ☐ ☐ ☐ ☐

Comments: _____

_____

_____

_____

_____

_____

_____

_____

_____

_____

"We lived on a diet when I was a kid. Some of our dinners were so small, I used to burp from memory." —Milton Berle

Day 74

Time	Amt.	Food	Cal.	Bal.	Fat Gm.	Bal.
		Ending Daily Balances				

Today's exercise   Duration

_____   _____

_____   _____

Calories burned _____

Check one box for each 8-oz. glass of water you drink

☐ ☐ ☐ ☐ ☐ ☐ ☐ ☐

Comments: _____

_____

_____

_____

_____

_____

_____

_____

_____

_____

"My wife is a light eater. As soon as it's light,
she starts eating." —Henny Youngman

Date _____

Day 75

Time	Amt.	Food	Cal.	Bal.	Fat Gm.	Bal.
		Ending Daily Balances				

Today's exercise   Duration

_____   _____

_____   _____

Calories burned _____

Check one box for each 8-oz. glass of water you drink

☐ ☐ ☐ ☐ ☐ ☐ ☐ ☐

Comments: _____

_____

_____

_____

_____

_____

_____

_____

_____

_____

Don't serve meals "family-style". Putting food in bowls
on the table tempts you to reach for second helpings.

Date _____

Day 76

Time	Amt.	Food	Cal.	Bal.	Fat Gm.	Bal.
		Ending Daily Balances				

Today's exercise	Duration
_____	_____
_____	_____

Calories burned _____

Check one box for each 8-oz. glass of water you drink

☐ ☐ ☐ ☐ ☐ ☐ ☐ ☐

Comments: _____

_____

_____

_____

_____

_____

_____

_____

_____

_____

My aunt knew she was in trouble when she went to the
department store and told the clerk, "I'd like to see a
bathing suit in my size" and the clerk replied, "So would I."

Date _____

Day 77

Time	Amt.	Food	Cal.	Bal.	Fat Gm.	Bal.
		Ending Daily Balances				

Today's exercise   Duration

_____   _____

_____   _____

Calories burned _____

Check one box for each 8-oz. glass of water you drink

☐ ☐ ☐ ☐ ☐ ☐ ☐ ☐

Comments: _____

_____

_____

_____

_____

_____

_____

_____

_____

_____

"Once during Prohibition, I was forced to live on nothing
but food and water for several days." —W.C. Fields

Date _____ **Day 78**

Time	Amt.	Food	Cal.	Bal.	Fat Gm.	Bal.
		Ending Daily Balances				

Today's exercise   Duration

_____   _____

_____   _____

Calories burned _____

Check one box for each 8-oz. glass of water you drink

☐ ☐ ☐ ☐ ☐ ☐ ☐ ☐

Comments: _____

_____

_____

_____

_____

_____

_____

_____

_____

_____

_____

Eleven weeks and still losing! Hurray! This
healthier eating could get to be a habit—one
that you can live with for a *loooong* time!

Date _____ **Day 79**

Time	Amt.	Food	Cal.	Bal.	Fat Gm.	Bal.
		Ending Daily Balances				

Today's exercise   Duration

_____   _____

_____   _____

Calories burned _____

Check one box for each 8-oz. glass of water you drink

☐   ☐   ☐   ☐   ☐   ☐   ☐   ☐

Comments: _____

_____

_____

_____

_____

_____

_____

_____

_____

_____

"The only reason I would take up jogging is so that I
could hear heavy breathing again." —Erma Bombeck

Date ——————

Day 80

Time	Amt.	Food	Cal.	Bal.	Fat Gm.	Bal.

Ending Daily Balances

Today's exercise   Duration

_____   _____

_____   _____

Calories burned _____

Check one box for each 8-oz. glass of water you drink

☐ ☐ ☐ ☐ ☐ ☐ ☐ ☐

Comments: _____

_____

_____

_____

_____

_____

_____

_____

_____

_____

_____

"I knew it was time to slow down on my eating when I started
putting whipped cream on my vitamin pills." —Jackie Gleason

Date _____

Day 81

Time	Amt.	Food	Cal.	Bal.	Fat Gm.	Bal.
		Ending Daily Balances				

Today's exercise   Duration

_____   _____

_____   _____

Calories burned _____

Check one box for each 8-oz. glass of water you drink

☐   ☐   ☐   ☐   ☐   ☐   ☐   ☐

Comments: _____

_____

_____

_____

_____

_____

_____

_____

_____

_____

Keep a support system for yourself. It's great to have some
friends join you on a walk or share low fat recipes with you.

Date _____ **Day 82**

Time	Amt.	Food	Cal.	Bal.	Fat Gm.	Bal.
		Ending Daily Balances				

Today's exercise   Duration

_____   _____

_____   _____

Calories burned _____

Check one box for each 8-oz. glass of water you drink

☐ ☐ ☐ ☐ ☐ ☐ ☐ ☐

Comments: _____

_____

_____

_____

_____

_____

_____

_____

_____

_____

"One can never consent to creep when one
feels an impulse to soar." —Helen Keller

Date —————— **Day 83**

Time	Amt.	Food	Cal.	Bal.	Fat Gm.	Bal.
		Ending Daily Balances				

Today's exercise   Duration

_____   _____

_____   _____

Calories burned _____

Check one box for each 8-oz. glass of water you drink

☐ ☐ ☐ ☐ ☐ ☐ ☐ ☐

Comments: _____

_____

_____

_____

_____

_____

_____

_____

_____

_____

"I have so many bad eating habits—the last time I
slurped soup in a restaurant, four couples got up to dance."
—Milton Berle

Date _____ **Day 84**

Time	Amt.	Food	Cal.	Bal.	Fat Gm.	Bal.
		Ending Daily Balances				

Today's exercise   Duration

_____   _____

_____   _____

Calories burned _____

Check one box for each 8-oz. glass of water you drink

☐   ☐   ☐   ☐   ☐   ☐   ☐   ☐

Comments: _____

_____

_____

_____

_____

_____

_____

_____

_____

_____

_____

Adding club soda to fruit juices adds sparkle, makes
them go farther, and reduces calories per portion.

Date ———————

Day 85

Time	Amt.	Food	Cal.	Bal.	Fat Gm.	Bal.
		Ending Daily Balances				

Today's exercise   Duration

_____   _____

_____   _____

Calories burned _____

Check one box for each 8-oz. glass of water you drink

☐ ☐ ☐ ☐ ☐ ☐ ☐ ☐

It's Weigh Day!

Starting weight _____ **Current weight** _____

_____ **pounds to lose until reaching 90-day goal.**

What's working? What's hindering? Revisions?

_____

_____

_____

_____

_____

_____

Just five more days to go!!!

Date _____

Day 86

Time	Amt.	Food	Cal.	Bal.	Fat Gm.	Bal.
		Ending Daily Balances				

Today's exercise   Duration

_____   _____

_____   _____

Calories burned _____

Check one box for each 8-oz. glass of water you drink

☐ ☐ ☐ ☐ ☐ ☐ ☐ ☐

Comments: _____

_____

_____

_____

_____

_____

_____

_____

_____

_____

"You know it's time to diet when you fall down and
rock yourself to sleep trying to get up." —Anonymous

Date _____

Day 87

Time	Amt.	Food	Cal.	Bal.	Fat Gm.	Bal.
Ending Daily Balances						

Today's exercise   Duration

_____   _____

_____   _____

           Calories burned _____

Check one box for each 8-oz. glass of water you drink

☐   ☐   ☐   ☐   ☐   ☐   ☐   ☐

Comments: _____

_____

_____

_____

_____

_____

_____

_____

_____

_____

"Quit worrying about your health—
eventually it will go away." —Anonymous

Date _____ **Day 88**

Time	Amt.	Food	Cal.	Bal.	Fat Gm.	Bal.
		Ending Daily Balances				

Today's exercise   Duration

_____   _____

_____   _____

Calories burned _____

Check one box for each 8-oz. glass of water you drink

☐ ☐ ☐ ☐ ☐ ☐ ☐ ☐

Comments: _____

_____

_____

_____

_____

_____

_____

_____

_____

_____

"Conscience is the small voice that keeps
interrupting when food is talking." —Anonymous

Date ———————

Day 89

Time	Amt.	Food	Cal.	Bal.	Fat Gm.	Bal.
		Ending Daily Balances				

Today's exercise   Duration

_____   _____

_____   _____

Calories burned _____

Check one box for each 8-oz. glass of water you drink

☐ ☐ ☐ ☐ ☐ ☐ ☐ ☐

Comments: _____

_____

_____

_____

_____

_____

_____

_____

_____

_____

"The most dangerous food of all is a wedding cake."
—American proverb

Day 90

Date _____

Time	Amount	Food	Calories	Bal.	Fat Gm.	Bal.
		Ending Daily Balances				

Today's exercise   Duration

_____   _____

_____   _____

Calories burned _____

Check one box for each 8-oz. glass of water you drink

☐   ☐   ☐   ☐   ☐   ☐   ☐   ☐

Final Weigh Day!

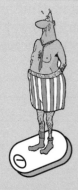

Starting weight _____ **Today's weight** _____

     I lost _____ pounds!!!!

Congratulations on a job well-done!
You can be proud of your accomplishment! If you
have more weight to lose, start another journal
and continue charting as you have been until
you reach your ultimate goal. On the following
pages review your past 90-day experience.

Describe the various problems that you encountered the past three months and the solutions you found to combat them. Write down how your emotions influenced your eating habits in the past and how you've learned to modify your responses to them in a healthier manner. What motivated you to stick with your regular exercise program? How do you feel differently about yourself? Do others respond differently to you? How has your health improved? What can you do now that you couldn't do before? Reviewing all of the positive changes that resulted from your weight loss will motivate you to get back on track if destructive eating habits begin to reappear.

Nutritional Values

Including Fast Foods!

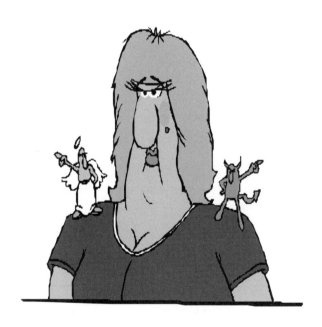

Let Your Conscience Be Your Guide!

Nutritional Information

Alcohol

Food Item	Amount	Fat Gm.	Calories
Beer			
regular	12 fl. oz.	0	150
light	12 fl. oz.	0	100
Champagne	6 fl. oz.	0	110
Cordials			
Amaretto	1 fl. oz.	0	100
Anisette	1 fl. oz.	0	100
B & B	1 fl. oz.	0	95
Benedictine	1 fl. oz.	0	95
Brandy (fruit flavored)	1 fl. oz.	0	95
Creme de Almonde	1 fl. oz.	0	100
Creme de Cacao	1 fl. oz.	0	100
Creme de Menthe	1 fl. oz.	0	125
Drambuie	1 fl. oz.	0	125
Peppermint Schnapps	1 fl. oz.	0	85
Sloe Gin	1 fl. oz.	0	85
Southern Comfort	1 fl. oz.	0	120
Tia Maria	1 fl. oz.	0	90
Triple Sec	1 fl. oz.	0	80
Liquor, Distilled (Note: the higher the proof, the higher the calories)			
80 proof	1 fl. oz.	0	65
86 proof	1 fl. oz.	0	70
90 proof	1 fl. oz.	0	75
94 proof	1 fl. oz.	0	80
100 proof	1 fl. oz.	0	85
Malt liquor	12 fl. oz.	0	190
Wine			
Burgundy	6 fl. oz.	0	130
Chablis	6 fl. oz.	0	120
Chardonnay	6 fl. oz.	0	120
Rosé	6 fl. oz.	0	130
Table wine, sweet	6 fl. oz.	0	270
White Zinfandel	6 fl. oz.	0	125
Wine cooler	8 fl. oz.	0	85

Beverages

Food Item	Amount	Fat Gm.	Calories
Club Soda	12 fl. oz.	0	0
Cocoa			
w/ skim milk	8 fl. oz.	2	160
w/ whole milk	8 fl. oz.	9	220
mix, no added sugar	1 serving	0	50
Coffee, brewed	8 fl. oz.	0	5
Coffee, flavored mixes, instant	6 fl. oz.	2	55
Crystal Light	8 fl. oz.	0	5
Eggnog	8 fl. oz.	20	350
Fruitopia, all flavors	8 fl. oz.	0	120
Gatorade	12 fl. oz.	0	90
Grape juice, canned	6 fl. oz.	0	120
Kool-Aid	8 fl. oz.	0	95
Lemonade	8 fl. oz.	0	100
Orange Juice, unsweetened	8 fl. oz.	0	110
Snapple			
iced tea	8 oz.	0	110
lemonade	8 oz.	0	110
Soft Drinks			
regular	12 fl. oz.	0	160
sugar-free	12 fl. oz.	0	0
Tang	8 fl. oz.	0	120
Tea	8 fl. oz.	0	0

Beverages (continued)

Food Item	Amount	Fat Gm.	Calories
Country Time Instant Tea	8 fl. oz.	0	70

Breads

Food Item	Amount	Fat Gm.	Calories
Bagel, plain	1 average	2	180
Biscuit			
baking powder	1 medium	7	160
buttermilk	1 medium	5	100
from mix	1 medium	4	120
Bisquick	1 cup	17	510
Bisquick, reduced fat	1 cup	8	450
Boboli shell	1/2	3	160
Breadsticks			
plain	1 stick	0	25
sesame	1 stick	4	30
Bread			
buttermilk	1 slice	1	70
French	1 slice	1	70
fruit	1 slice	3	120
honey wheat	1 slice	1	70
Italian	1 slice	1	80
"lite" varieties	1 slice	1	40
multi-grain	1 slice	1	70
pita, plain	1 large	1	240
pita, whole wheat	1 large	1	200
raisin	1 slice	1	70
Roman Meal	1 slice	1	70
rye, American	1 slice	1	70
rye, pumpernickel	1 slice	1	80
sourdough	1 slice	1	70
white, enriched	1 slice	1	70
whole wheat	1 slice	1	60
bread crumbs, dry	1 cup	5	400
Coffee cake	1 piece	8	220
Cornbread	1 slice	8	200
Cornmeal	1 cup	2	500
Cornstarch	1 T.	0	35
Crackers			
cheese	5 pieces	5	80
Cheese Nips	10 crackers	3	60
Cheese Nips, Air Crisps	32 crackers	4	130
cheese w/ peanut butter	2 oz. pkg.	13	280
Goldfish	15 crackers	2	40
graham	4 squares	2	120
graham, low fat	12 squares	2	165
Harvest Wheats	5 crackers	4	90
Hi Ho	5 crackers	5	100
melba toast	1 piece	0	15
oyster	20 crackers	2	80
rice cakes	1 cake	0	35
Ritz	5 crackers	5	85
Ritz, reduced fat	8 crackers	4	110
Ritz Bits	23 pieces	5	85
Ritz Cheese	4 crackers	5	100
Rye Krisp	2 crackers	0	50
Saltines	2 crackers	1	26
Fat-free saltines	5 crackers	0	50
Snackwell Wheat	5 crackers	0	60
Sociables	6 crackers	3	70
soda	6 crackers	2	50
Tater Crisps, Mr. Phipps	22 crackers	4	130

Nutritional Information

Food Item	Amount	Fat Gm.	Calories
Breads (continued)			
Triscuit	3 crackers	2	65
Triscuit, reduced fat	4 crackers	2	65
Wasa crispbread	1 piece	1	45
Waverly Wafers	3 crackers	2	50
Wheat Thins	5 crackers	2	45
Wheat Thins, reduced fat	18 crackers	3	130
Wheatsworth	5 crackers	3	70
Zwieback	3 crackers	1	60
Crepe	1 large	2	60
Croissant	1 medium	11	160
Croutons	1/4 cup	2	45
Danish	1 medium	20	250
Doughnut, cake	1 average	18	250
English muffin	1	1	135
Flour			
rice	1 cup	1	430
soy	1 cup	18	380
white	1 cup	1	400
white, all purpose	1 cup	1	420
whole wheat	1 cup	2	400
French toast			
frozen	1 slice	6	140
homemade	1 slice	10	170
Hushpuppy	1 average	11	150
Matzo ball	1	8	125
Muffins, most varieties	1 large	15	300
banana nut	1 medium	5	135
Betty Crocker, fat-free	1 medium	0	110
blueberry, from mix	1 medium	4	125
bran, homemade	1 medium	5	110
corn	1 medium	4	130
Krusteaz, fat-free blueberry	1 medium	0	130
Pancakes			
blueberry, (mix)	3 medium	15	320
buckwheat (mix)	3 medium	12	270
buttermilk (mix)	3 medium	10	270
homemade	3 medium	10	300
"lite" (mix)	3 medium	2	130
Popover	1	5	170
Pop-tarts, mini, frosted chocolate	1 pouch	4	170
Pop-tarts, low fat	1	3	190
Rolls			
brown & serve	1	2	90
cloverleaf	1	3	90
crescent	1	6	100
croissant	1 medium	8	135
French	1	1	140
hamburger	1	3	180
hard	1	1	120
hot dog	1	2	120
kaiser/hoagie	1 large	2	180
parkerhouse	1	2	60
rye	1	2	55
sesame seed	1	2	60
submarine	1 large	5	400
wheat	1	2	60
white	1	2	110
white, homemade	1	3	120
whole wheat	1	1	85
Scone	1	6	130

Food Item	Amount	Fat Gm.	Calories
Breads (continued)			
Stuffing			
bread, mix	1/2 cup	12	200
corn bread, mix	1/2 cup	5	175
Stove Top	1/2 cup	9	175
Sweet roll, iced	1 medium	8	200
Tortilla			
corn, 8"	1	3	70
flour, 8"	1	5	90
Turnover, fruit filled	1	20	225
Waffle			
frozen	1 medium	4	100
frozen, Aunt Jemima low fat	2	1	160
homemade	1 large	13	245

Candy

Butterscotch	8 pieces	3	140
Butterscotch chips	1 oz.	7	230
Candied fruit	1 oz.	0	90
Candy bars			
Almond Joy	1 oz.	8	130
Baby Ruth	1 oz.	7	140
Bit-o-Honey	1 oz.	2	120
Butterfinger	1 oz.	6	130
Chunky, milk chocolate	1 oz.	4	120
Chunky, original	1 oz.	7	140
Crunch'n Munch, reduced fat	1 cup	4	210
Golden Almond, Hershey	1 oz.	11	150
Heath	1 oz.	9	150
Kit Kat	1 oz.	8	150
Krackle, Hershey	1 oz.	7	135
Mars	1 oz.	7	135
milk chocolate, w/ almonds	1 oz.	10	150
milk chocolate, Hershey	1 oz.	9	150
milk chocolate, Nestle	1 oz.	9	145
Milky Way	1 oz.	4	120
Milky Way Lite	1.57 oz. bar	5	170
Mounds	1 oz.	7	130
Mr. Goodbar	1 oz.	11	155
Nestle's Crunch	1 oz.	8	150
Peppermint patty, York	1.5 oz. patty	4	170
Snickers	1 oz.	7	135
Special Dark, Hershey	1 oz.	9	150
Three Musketeers	1 oz.	4	140
Twix	1 oz.	7	140
Cadbury Creme Eggs	1 oz.	6	140
Candy-coated almonds	1 oz.	5	130
Caramel corn	1 cup	7	150
Caramel w/o nuts	1 oz.	6	115
Chocolate chips			
Hershey's reduced fat	1 oz.	7	120
milk chocolate	1/4 cup	11	220
semi-sweet	1/4 cup	12	220
Chocolate-covered cherries	1 oz.	5	125
Chocolate-covered cream center	1 oz.	5	125
Chocolate-covered peanuts	1 oz.	12	160
Chocolate-covered raisins	1 oz.	5	120
Candy Kisses	6 pieces	9	150
Chocolate Stars	6 pieces	7	140
English Toffee	1 oz.	3	110
Fudge w/ marshmallows	1 oz.	2	90

Nutritional Information

Food Item	Amount	Fat Gm.	Calories
Candy (continued)			
Fudge w/o nuts	1 oz.	3	110
Fudge w/ nuts	1 oz.	5	120
Good & Plenty	1 oz.	0	105
Gumdrops	30	0	100
Hard candy	5 pieces	0	100
Jelly beans	1 oz.	0	100
Licorice	1 oz.	0	35
Life Savers	6	0	50
M&Ms, plain	1 oz.	6	130
M&Ms, peanut	1 oz.	8	145
Malted milk balls	1 oz.	7	140
Marshmallow	1	0	25
Mints	20	1	150
Peanut brittle	1 oz.	9	150
Reese's Peanut Butter Cup	1	9	150
Sugar Daddy	1 oz.	1	150
Taffy	1 oz.	1	100
Tootsie Roll	1 oz.	2	110
Cereals			
All Bran	1 cup	1	215
Alpha-Bits	1 cup	1	110
Apple Jacks	1 cup	0	110
Bran Buds	1 cup	2	200
Bran Chex	1 cup	1	135
Bran Flakes 40%	1 cup	1	125
Bran, 100%	1 cup	4	200
Brown Sugar Sq., Healthy Choice	1 cup	1	155
Cap'n Crunch	1 cup	4	160
Cheerios	1 cup	2	90
Corn Chex	1 cup	0	110
Cornflakes	1 cup	0	110
Cracklin Oat Bran	1 cup	8	200
Cream of Wheat	1 cup	0	140
Fiber One	1 cup	2	130
Fruit Loops	1 cup	0	110
Fruit & Fiber w/ apples & cinn.	1 cup	0	180
Fruit & Fiber w/ dts., rsn., & wlnts.	1 cup	2	180
Golden Grahams	1 cup	1	135
Granola	1 cup	15	400
Kellogg's low fat granola	1 cup	6	360
Grapenut Flakes	1 cup	0	115
Grapenuts	1 cup	0	420
Honeynut Cheerios	1 cup	1	135
Kix	1 cup	0	75
Life	1 cup	0	160
Nut 'n Honey	1 cup	2	165
Nutri-Grain	1 cup	1	135
Oat bran, cooked	1 cup	2	110
Oats, instant	1 packet	2	110
Peanut Butter Puffs, Reese's	1 cup	4	175
Product 19	1 cup	0	110
Puffed Rice	1 cup	0	60
Puffed Wheat	1 cup	0	45
Raisin Bran	1 cup	1	155
Raisin Squares	1 cup	1	240
Rice Chex	1 cup	0	110
Rice Krispies	1 cup	0	110
Shredded Wheat	1 cup	0	85
Shredded Wheat Squares,frt.-fld.	1 cup	0	180

Food Item	Amount	Fat Gm.	Calories
Cereals (continued)			
Special K	1 cup	0	110
Sugar Frosted Flakes	1 cup	0	150
Sugar Smacks	1 cup	1	130
Team	1 cup	1	110
Wheat Chex	1 cup	1	170
Wheaties	1 cup	1	100
Cheese			
Alpine Lace, Free 'n Lean			
American	1 oz.	0	35
Cheddar	1 oz.	0	35
Mozzarella	1 oz.	0	35
American			
light	1 oz.	4	70
processed	1 oz.	9	105
Blue	1 oz.	8	100
Brick	1 oz.	8	105
Brie	1 oz.	8	95
Caraway	1 oz.	8	110
Cheddar	1 oz.	9	115
Cheddar, reduced fat	1 oz.	6	90
Cheese food, cold pack	2 T.	8	95
Cheese sauce	1/2 cup	20	260
Cheese spread, Kraft	1 oz.	6	80
Cheez Whiz	1 oz.	6	80
Colby	1 oz.	9	110
Cottage Cheese			
fat-free	1/2 cup	0	90
1 % fat	1/2 cup	1	80
2 % fat	1/2 cup	2	100
creamed	1/2 cup	5	120
Cream Cheese			
Kraft-free	2 T.	0	25
"lite" Neufchatel	2 T.	0	75
regular	1 oz.	10	100
Weight Watchers	1 oz.	2	35
Edam	1 oz.	8	100
Feta	1 oz.	6	75
Gouda	1 oz.	8	100
Healthy Choice (chunk)	1 oz.	0	40
Hot Pepper	1 oz.	7	90
Jarlsberg	1 oz.	7	100
Kraft American Singles	1 oz.	7	90
Kraft Free	1 oz.	0	45
Kraft Light 'n Lively	1 oz.	4	70
Limburger	1 oz.	8	95
Monterey Jack	1 oz.	9	110
Mozzarella			
part skim	1 oz.	5	75
whole milk	1 oz.	6	80
whole milk, low moisture	1 oz.	7	90
Muenster	1 oz.	9	105
Parmesan			
grated	1 T.	2	25
hard	1 oz.	7	110
Port wine, cold pack	1 oz.	9	100
Provolone	1 oz.	8	100
Ricotta			
"lite" reduced fat	1/2 cup	4	110
part skim	1/2 cup	10	170

Nutritional Information

Food Item	Amount	Fat Gm.	Calories
Cheese (continued)			
whole milk	1/2 cup	16	215
Romano	1 oz.	8	110
Roquefort	1 oz.	9	105
Smoked cheese product	1 oz.	7	90
Swiss			
aged	1 oz.	8	110
processed	1 oz.	7	95
Velveeta Light	1 oz.	4	70

Desserts & Toppings

Food Item	Amount	Fat Gm.	Calories
Apple Betty, fruit crisps	1/2 cup	13	340
Baklava	1 piece	29	425
Brownie			
chocolate, plain	1 small	3	60
chocolate w/ walnuts & icing	1 medium	5	60
Hostess	1 small	6	150
Little Debbie, chocolate	1 small	4	110
Pepperidge Farm	1	9	170
Snackwell brownie	1	2	130
Cake			
angel food	1/12 cake	0	160
banana w/ frosting	1/12 cake	16	390
black forest	1/12 cake	14	280
butter w/ frosting	1/12 cake	13	380
carrot w/ frosting	1/12 cake	19	420
chocolate w/ frosting	1/12 cake	17	390
chocolate, Betty Crocker lite	1/10 cake	3	230
coconut w/ frosting	1/12 cake	18	395
German chocolate w/ frosting	1/12 cake	18	400
gingerbread	2 1/2 " slice	3	270
lemon chiffon	1/12 cake	4	190
lemon w/ frosting	1/12 cake	13	360
marble w/ frosting	1/12 cake	16	410
pineapple upside-down	2 1/2 " slice	9	240
pound	1/12 cake	9	200
pound, Entenmann fat-free	1 oz. slice	0	70
shortbread w/ fruit	1 piece	9	345
spice w/ frosting	1/12 cake	11	325
sponge	1 piece	3	195
Sweet Rewards	1/8 cake	0	170
white w/ frosting	1/12 cake	14	370
yellow w/ frosting	1/12 cake	16	390
Cheesecake	1/8 pie	22	370
Cobbler			
w/ biscuit topping	1/2 cup	6	210
w/ pie crust topping	1/2 cup	9	235
Cookies			
animal crackers	15 cookies	3	120
Bordeaux, Pepperidge Farm	1	2	40
Capri, Pepperidge Farm	1	5	80
Chips Ahoy, reduced fat	3	6	150
Chips Deluxe, Keebler, red. fat	1	3	70
chocolate	1	3	55
chocolate chip, homemade	1	4	70
chocolate chip, Pepperidge Farm	1 large	7	160
fig bar	1	1	55
fudge cookie cakes, Snackwell	1	0	50
Gingersnap	1	2	35
Graham cracker, chocolate cvrd.	1	3	60
Lemon Nut, Pepperidge Farm	1 large	9	170

Food Item	Amount	Fat Gm.	Calories
Desserts & Toppings (continued)			
Macaroon, coconut	1	2	50
Milano, Pepperidge Farm	1	4	60
Molasses	1	2	70
Oatmeal	1	3	80
Oatmeal raisin	1	3	80
Oatmeal, Pepperidge Farm	1	6	155
Oreo	1	2	50
reduced fat	3	5	140
Orleans, Pepperidge Farm	1	2	30
Peanut butter	1	3	70
Rice Krispie bar	1	1	35
Shortbread	1	2	40
Snackwell cream sandwiches	1	1	55
Sugar	1	3	90
Sugar wafers	2 small	2	55
Tea biscuit	1	1	20
Teddy Graham s, Nabisco	25	4	140
Vanilla creme sandwich, regular	1	3	70
Vanilla creme sndw, Snackwell's	3	4	165
Vanilla Wafers	3	2	50
Vienna Finger, Sunshine, red.	3	5	195
Cream Puff	1	15	245
Creamsicle	1 bar	3	105
Cupcake			
chocolate w/ icing	1	5	160
yellow w/ icing	1	6	160
Custard, baked	1/2 cup	7	150
Date bar	1 bar	3	95
Dreamsicle	1 bar	6	205
Dumpling, fruit	1 piece	15	325
Eclair			
w/ chocolate icing & custard	1 small	15	315
w/ chocolate icing & whipped cr.	1 small	26	295
Frosting			
chocolate	3 T.	5	150
cream cheese	3 T.	7	170
lemon	3 T,	4	140
ready-to-spread	1/2 tube	7	170
seven-minute	3 T.	0	135
vanilla	3 T.	4	140
Fruitcake	1 piece	6	155
Fudgesicle	1 bar	0	195
Gelatin			
low cal.	1/2 cup	0	10
regular	1/2 cup	0	70
Granola bar	1 bar	6	140
Hostess products			
Cupcake	1	7	205
Ding Dong	1	9	170
Fruit Snack Pie	1	20	400
Ho Ho	1	7	135
Honey Bun	1	33	570
Snoball	1	4	150
Twinkie	1	4	145
Ice cream bar			
chocolate coated	1 bar	11	180
toffee crunch	1 bar	10	150
Ice cream cake roll	1 slice	7	160
Ice cream cone (cone only)	1 medium	0	45
Ice cream drumstick	1	10	190

Nutritional Information

Food Item	Amount	Fat Gm.	Calories
Desserts & Toppings (continued)			
Ice cream sandwich	1	6	170
Ice cream			
chocolate	1/2 cup	7	135
chocolate gourmet	1/2 cup	12	175
fat-free	1/2 cup	0	110
French vanilla soft serve	1/2 cup	11	185
strawberry	1/2 cup	6	130
vanilla	1/2 cup	7	135
vanilla, Häagen-Dazs	1/2 cup	17	250
Weight Watchers (1% fat)	1/2 cup	9	80
Ice Milk			
chocolate	1/2 cup	3	90
soft serve, all flavors	1/2 cup	2	110
strawberry	1/2 cup	2	105
vanilla	1/2 cup	3	90
Ladyfinger	1	2	80
Lemon bars	1 bar	3	70
Mousse, chocolate	1/2 cup	15	190
Napoleon	1 piece	5	85
Pie			
apple	1/8 pie	17	350
banana cream or custard	1/8 pie	14	355
blueberry	1/8 pie	17	385
Boston cream pie	1/8 pie	8	260
cherry	1/8 pie	18	420
chocolate cream	1/8 pie	13	310
chocolate meringue	1/8 pie	18	380
coconut cream or custard	1/8 pie	19	365
key lime	1/8 pie	19	390
lemon chiffon	1/8 pie	13	335
lemon meringue	1/8 pie	12	320
mincemeat	1/8 pie	18	435
peach	1/8 pie	17	420
pecan	1/8 pie	23	510
pumpkin	1/8 pie	17	365
raisin	1/8 pie	13	325
rhubarb	1/8 pie	17	405
strawberry	1/8 pie	9	230
sweet potato	1/8 pie	18	340
Pie tart, fruit filled	1 pie	19	360
Popsicle			
Kemps sugar-free	1	0	5
regular	1	0	95
Pudding			
most flavors	1/2 cup	5	170
bread	1/2 cup	8	220
chocolate w/ whole milk	1/2 cup	9	245
D-Zerta lo-cal w/ skim milk	1/2 cup	0	65
D-Zerta lo-cal w/ whole milk	1/2 cup	0	95
pistachio, sugar-free	1/2 cup	0	70
rice	1/2 cup	6	180
tapioca	1/2 cup	5	125
Pudding Pop, frozen	1	2	75
Sherbet	1/2 cup	2	135
Souffle, chocolate	1/2 cup	4	65
Strudel, fruit	1/2 cup	1	50
Tasty Kake			
butterscotch Krimpet	1	2	120
chocolate junior	1	12	305
coconut cream	1	31	480

Food Item	Amount	Fat Gm.	Calories
Desserts & Toppings (continued)			
fruit pie	1	14	360
jelly Krimpet	1	1	95
Toppings			
butterscotch, caramel	3 T.	0	155
chocolate fudge	2 T.	4	100
chocolate syrup, Hershey	2 T.	0	70
marshmallow creme	3 T.	0	160
milk chocolate fudge	2 T.	5	120
Mrs. Richardson's			
butterscotch	2 T.	1	130
caramel, fat-free	2 T.	0	130
hot fudge, fat-free	2 T.	0	110
pineapple	3 T.	0	145
strawberry	3 T.	0	140
whipped topping			
aerosol	1/4 cup	4	45
frozen	1/4 cup	4	80
non-dairy lite	1/4 cup	2	30
whipping cream			
heavy, fluid	1 T.	6	50
light, fluid	1 T.	5	45
Turnover, fruit filled	1	19	225
Yogurt, frozen			
low fat	1/2 cup	3	110
non fat	1/2 cup	0	80

Eggs

Food Item	Amount	Fat Gm.	Calories
Boiled/poached	1	6	80
Fried w. 1/2 T. fat	1	10	110
Omelet			
plain, 3 egg	1	21	270
Denver, 3 egg	1	26	300
Scrambled with milk	1	8	100
Substitute, Egg Beaters	1/4 cup	0	30
White	1	0	15
Yolk	1	6	65

Fish (all baked w/o added fat)

Food Item	Amount	Fat Gm.	Calories
Abalone, canned	3 oz.	0	85
Anchovy, canned	3 fillets	1	20
Bass			
freshwater	3 oz.	3	90
striped	3 oz.	3	90
Catfish	3 oz.	3	90
Clams			
canned, solids & liquid	1/2 cup	1	50
canned, solids only	3 oz.	2	125
meat only	5 large	1	80
soft, raw	4 large	2	60
Cod			
canned	3 oz.	0	75
cooked	3 oz.	0	70
Crab			
Alaskan King	3 oz.	1	85
cake	3 oz.	9	155
canned	1/2 cup	2	85
deviled	3 oz.	9	175
fried	3 oz.	16	230
Crappie	3 oz.	1	70
Flounder	3 oz.	0	60

Nutritional Information

Food Item	Amount	Fat Gm.	Calories
Fish(continued)			
Gefilte	3 oz.	2	70
Grouper	3 oz.	1	75
Haddock			
baked	3 oz.	1	70
fried	3 oz.	9	155
smoked/canned	3 oz.	0	90
Halibut	3 oz.	2	90
Herring			
canned or smoked	3 oz.	11	180
cooked	3 oz.	9	150
pickled	3 oz.	15	235
Lake trout	3 oz.	17	200
Lobster, northern			
boiled	3 oz.	2	80
broiled w/ fat	12 oz.	24	310
Mackerel			
Atlantic	3 oz.	12	190
Pacific	3 oz.	7	160
Muskie	3 oz.	2	95
Mussels			
canned	3 oz.	3	100
raw	3 oz.	2	75
Ocean perch			
baked	3 oz.	2	100
fried	3 oz.	10	185
Octopus	3 oz.	1	70
Oysters			
canned	3 oz.	2	60
fried	3 oz.	10	170
raw	6 medium	2	60
Perch	3 oz.	1	80
Pickerel	3 oz.	0	75
Pike			
northern	3 oz.	1	80
walleye	3 oz.	1	80
Pollock	3 oz.	1	80
Red snapper	3 oz.	2	80
Roughy, orange	3 oz.	6	110
Salmon			
Atlantic	3 oz.	5	120
baked/broiled	3 oz.	6	150
chinook, canned	3 oz.	12	180
pink, canned	3 oz.	5	105
smoked	3 oz.	8	150
Sardines	3 oz.	8	135
Scallops			
cooked	3 oz.	1	70
fried	3 oz.	9	170
steamed	3 oz.	1	90
Sea bass	3 oz.	1	80
Shrimp			
canned	3 oz.	3	155
fried	3 oz.	10	200
raw	3 oz.	1	90
Smelt, canned	4-5 med.	13	200
Sole	3 oz.	0	60
Squid			
fried	3 oz.	6	150
raw	3 oz.	1	110
Sushi	3 oz.	4	120

Food Item	Amount	Fat Gm.	Calories
Fish (continued)			
Swordfish	3 oz.	4	100
Trout			
brook	3 oz.	2	85
rainbow	3 oz.	9	165
Tuna			
bluefin, raw	3 oz.	4	120
light, canned in oil	3 oz.	20	230
canned in water	3 oz.	1	100
white, canned in oil	3 oz.	20	230
white, canned in water	3 oz.	1	100
yellowfin raw	3 oz.	1	90
White perch	3 oz.	3	100
Yellowtail	3 oz.	5	120
Fruit			
Apple			
dried	1/2 cup	0	155
fresh	1 medium	0	80
Applesauce, unsweetened	1/2 cup	0	50
Apricots			
dried	5 halves	0	80
fresh	3 medium	0	50
Avocado	1	29	325
Banana	1 medium	1	105
Blackberries			
fresh	1 cup	0	75
frozen, unsweetened	1 cup	1	100
Blueberries			
fresh	1 cup	1	80
frozen, unsweetened	1 cup	1	80
Boysenberries, frzn. unswtned.	1 cup	0	65
Cantaloupe	1 cup	0	60
Cherries			
fresh	1/2 cup	1	50
maraschino	1/4 cup	0	55
sour, canned in heavy syrup	1/2 cup	0	115
Cranberries, fresh	1 cup	0	45
Cranberry sauce	1/2 cup	0	210
Cranberry-orange relish	1/2 cup	1	245
Crasins	1/4 cup	0	100
Dates, whole, dried	1/2 cup	0	230
Figs			
canned	3 figs	0	75
dried, uncooked	10 figs	1	475
fresh	1 medium	0	40
Fruit cocktail, canned w/ juice	1 cup	0	110
Fruit Roll-Up	1	1	50
Grapes, Thompson seedless	1/2 cup	0	95
Grapefruit	1/2 medium	0	40
Guava	1 medium	0	45
Honeydew melon	1/4 small	0	30
Kiwi	1 medium	0	50
Kumquat	1 medium	0	10
Lemon	1 medium	0	20
Lime	1 medium	0	20
Mandarin oranges, canned	1/2 cup	0	50
Mango	1 medium	1	135
Melon balls,	1 cup	0	55
Mixed fruit			
dried	1/2 cup	1	250

Nutritional Information

Food Item	Amount	Fat Gm.	Calories
Fruits (continued)			
Mixed fruit, frozen, sweetened	1 cup	1	245
Nectarine	1 medium	1	70
Orange	1 medium	0	60
Papaya	1 medium	0	120
Peach			
canned in heavy syrup	1 cup	0	190
canned in light syrup	1 cup	0	135
canned, water pack	1 cup	0	60
fresh	1 medium	0	40
Pear			
canned in heavy syrup	1 cup	0	190
canned in light syrup	1 cup	0	145
fresh	1 medium	1	100
Persimmon	1 medium	0	30
Pineapple			
canned in syrup	1 cup	2	190
canned, unsweetened	1 cup	0	140
fresh	1 cup	1	80
Plum			
canned in heavy syrup	1/2 cup	0	120
fresh	1 medium	1	35
Pomegranate	1 medium	0	100
Prunes, dried cooked	1/2 cup	0	110
Raisins	1/4 cup	0	110
Raspberries			
fresh	1 cup	0	60
frozen, sweetened	1 cup	0	105
Rhubarb	1 cup	0	25
Strawberries			
fresh	1 cup	0	45
frozen, sweetened	1 cup	0	245
frozen, unsweetened	1 cup	0	50
Tangerine	1 medium	0	35
Watermelon	1 cup	0	50
Fruit/Veg. Juices			
Apple cider	1 cup	0	120
Apple juice	1 cup	0	115
Apricot juice	1 cup	0	125
Carrot juice	1 cup	0	80
Cranberry juice cocktail			
low cal	1 cup	0	45
regular	1 cup	0	150
Cranberry-apple juice	1 cup	0	130
Grape juice	1 cup	0	155
Grapefruit juice	1 cup	0	95
Hawaiian Punch, regular	6 oz.	0	90
Hi-C	6 oz.	0	95
Lemon juice	2 T.	0	10
Lime juice	2 T.	0	10
Orange juice	1 cup	0	110
Orange-grapefruit juice	1 cup	0	110
Peach nectar	1 cup	0	135
Pear nectar	1 cup	0	150
Pineapple juice	1 cup	0	140
Pineapple-orange juice	1 cup	0	125
Prune juice	1 cup	0	180
Raspberry juice	1 cup	0	120
Tomato juice	1 cup	0	40
V-8 juice	1 cup	0	50

Food Item	Amount	Fat Gm.	Calories
Gravies, Sauces, & Dips			
Au Jus, mix	1 cup	0	50
Barbecue sauce	1 T.	0	10
Bearnaise sauce, mix	1/4 package	25	265
Brown Gravy			
beef, Heinz fat-free	1/4 cup	0	15
canned	1/2 can	3	80
from mix	1/2 cup	0	30
homemade	1/4 cup	14	165
Catsup	1 T.	0	15
Chicken Gravy			
canned	1/2 can	8	120
from mix	1/2 cup	1	40
giblet from can	1/4 cup	2	35
Pepperidge Farm, 98% fat-free	1/4 cup	1	25
Chili sauce	1 T.	0	15
Cocktail sauce	2 T.	0	25
Dip, sour cream based	2 T.	5	50
Guacamole dip	1 oz.	12	110
Hollandaise sauce	1/4 cup	18	180
Horseradish sauce, Kraft	1 T.	2	20
Home-style gravy, mix	1/4 cup	1	25
Mushroom gravy			
canned	1/2 can	4	75
from mix	1/2 cup	1	35
Mushroom sauce, from mix	1/4 package	3	70
Mustard			
brown	1 T.	1	15
yellow	1 T.	1	10
Onion dip	2 T.	4	60
Onion gravy, mix	1/2 cup	1	40
Pesto sauce, commercial	1 oz.	15	155
Picante sauce	6 T.	1	50
Pork gravy, mix	1/2 cup	1	40
Sour cream sauce	1/4 cup	12	125
Soy sauce	1 T.	0	10
Soy sauce, reduced sodium	1 T.	0	10
Spaghetti sauce			
canned, w/o meat	1/2 cup	4	80
Healthy Choice, extra chunky	1/2 cup	5	50
homemade w/ meat	1/2 cup	18	240
Pasta Toss, Ragu	1/2 cup	8	120
Prego w/ mushrooms	1/2 cup	6	135
Prego w/ meat flavor	1/2 cup	6	140
Ragu, extra chunky	1/2 cup	6	120
Ranch dip	1 T.	1	30
Spinach dip	2 T.	7	75
Steak sauce	1 T.	0	10
Stir fry sauce	1 T.	1	30
Stroganoff sauce, mix	1/4 pkg.	3	75
Sweet & sour sauce	1/4 pkg.	0	130
Tabasco sauce	1 T.	0	6
Taco sauce	1 T.	0	7
Tartar sauce	1 T.	8	70
fat-free	1 T.	0	25
Teriyaki sauce	1 T.	0	15
Turkey gravy			
canned	1/2 can	3	75
mix	1/2 can	1	40
White sauce	1/2 cup	12	220
Worcestershire sauce	1 T.	0	10

Nutritional Information

Food Item	Amount	Fat Gm.	Calories
Meats (all cooked w/o fat unless noted)			
Beef (extra lean, 7.5-12.4% fat)	3 oz.	8	170
arm/blade pot roast	3 oz.	8	170
club steak, lean	3 oz.	11	205
flank steak, fat trimmed	3 oz.	7	165
hindshank, lean	3 oz.	8	180
Liver			
braised	3 oz.	4	135
fried	3 oz.	7	185
porterhouse steak, lean	3 oz.	9	200
rib steak, lean	3 oz.	8	180
round			
bottom, lean	3 oz.	8	180
eye of round, lean	3 oz.	4	110
rump, lean, pot roasted	3 oz.	6	155
top, lean	3 oz.	5	180
sirloin steak, lean	3 oz.	8	170
sirloin steak, lean & fat	3 oz.	16	240
sirloin tip, lean, roasted	3 oz.	8	175
tenderloin, lean, broiled	3 oz.	10	190
top sirloin, lean, broiled	3 oz.	7	170
Beef, extra lean, approx. 15% fat	3 oz.	13	225
chuck, separable lean	3 oz.	13	225
cubed steak	3 oz.	13	225
hamburger			
extra lean	3 oz.	12	215
drained and rinsed	3 oz.	7	190
rib roast, lean	3 oz.	7	190
sirloin tips, roasted	3 oz.	13	225
stew meat, round, raw	3 oz.	12	225
T-bone, lean only	3 oz.	9	200
tenderloin, marbled	3 oz.	13	225
Beef, lean, approx. 20% fat	3 oz.	17	245
chuck, ground	3 oz.	20	285
hamburger, regular	3 oz.	17	245
meatballs	3 oz.	15	210
porterhouse steak, marbled	3 oz.	17	245
rib steak	3 oz.	13	245
rump, pot roast	3 oz.	17	245
short ribs, lean only	3 oz.	17	245
sirloin, broiled	3 oz.	16	245
Beef, regular, approx. 25% fat	3 oz.	23	305
arm/blade, pot roast	3 oz.	23	305
brisket, lean and marbled	3 oz.	26	315
chuck, stew meat	3 oz.	30	365
corned, medium fat	3 oz.	26	315
rib roast	3 oz.	26	315
ribeye steak, marbled	3 oz.	33	380
short ribs	3 oz.	27	320
sirloin, ground	3 oz.	23	305
steak, chicken fried	3 oz.	26	320
T-bone, broiled	3 oz.	23	305
Lamb			
blade chop,			
lean	3 oz.	6	128
lean and fat	3 oz.	22	325
leg			
lean	3 oz.	7	155
lean and fat	3 oz.	12	220
loin chop			
lean	3 oz.	7	155

Food Item	Amount	Fat Gm.	Calories
Meats (continued)			
lean and fat	3 oz.	18	260
rib chop			
lean	3 oz.	7	155
lean and fat	3 oz.	18	250
shoulder			
lean	3 oz.	9	215
lean and fat	3 oz.	23	370
Miscellaneous meats			
bacon substitute, strip	2 strips	4	50
beefalo	3 oz.	5	160
frog legs			
cooked	4 large	1	70
flour-coated and fried	6 large	29	420
rabbit, stewed	3 oz.	9	185
tongue	1 oz.	6	75
venison, roasted	3 oz.	2	135
Pork			
bacon			
cured, broiled	1 slice	3	35
cured, raw	1 slice	16	155
bacon bits	1 T.	1	20
blade			
lean	3 oz.	9	190
lean and fat	3 oz.	15	250
butt			
lean	3 oz.	12	260
lean and fat	3 oz.	24	295
Canadian bacon, broiled	1 oz.	2	40
Ham			
cured, butt, lean	3 oz.	4	140
cured, butt, lean and fat	3 oz.	11	210
cured, canned	3 oz.	5	120
cured, shank, lean	3 oz.	5	150
cured, shank, lean and fat	2 slices	14	255
fresh, lean	3 oz.	5	190
fresh, lean and fat	3 oz.	15	265
ham loaf, glazed	3 oz.	13	210
loin chop			
lean	3 oz.	7	170
lean and fat	3 oz.	14	295
smoked	3 oz.	9	150
smoked, 95% lean	3 oz.	5	125
picnic			
cured, lean	3 oz.	9	180
fresh, lean	3 oz.	6	130
shoulder, lean	2 slices	5	160
shoulder, marbled	2 slices	14	235
pig's feet, pickled	1 oz.	4	55
rib chop, trimmed	3 oz.	9	180
rib roast, trimmed	3 oz.	9	175
sausage			
brown and serve	1 oz.	9	105
link	1/2 oz.	5	50
patty	1 oz.	8	100
sirloin, lean, roasted	3 oz.	9	175
spareribs, roasted	6 medium	35	395
tenderloin, lean, roast	3 oz.	4	135
top loin chop, trimmed	3 oz.	7	165
Processed meats			
bacon substitute	2 strips	4	50

Nutritional Information

Food Item	Amount	Fat Gm.	Calories
Meats (continued)			
beef breakfast strips	2 strips	7	115
beef jerky	1 oz.	4	110
beef, chipped	2 slices	3	115
bologna, beef and pork	1 oz.	8	85
bratwurst			
pork	3 oz. link	33	380
pork and beef	3 oz. link	29	340
turkey	3 oz. link	10	160
braunschweiger	1 oz.	8	65
corn dog	1	20	330
corned beef	3 oz.	9	95
ham, chopped	1 oz.	2	55
ham, Louis Rich Carving Board	3 slices	2	75
hot dog			
beef or pork	1	13	145
chicken	1	9	115
Healthy Choice	2	3	100
Hormel 97% fat-free	1	1	45
turkey	1	8	100
kielbasa (Polish sausage)	1 oz.	8	80
knockwurst, knackwurst	2 oz. link	19	210
liver pâté, goose	1 oz.	12	130
Lunchables			
ham & cheddar	1 pkg.	22	360
low fat ham & swiss combo	1 pkg.	10	360
pepperoni	1 oz.	13	150
pork and beef	1 oz.	9	100
salami			
cooked	1 oz.	10	115
dry/hard	1 oz.	10	125
sausage			
Italian, mild or hot	2 oz. link	17	215
Polish	1 oz. link	8	90
smoked	2 oz. link	20	230
Vienna	1 sausage	4	45
Spam	1 oz.	7	90
Turkey ham	3 oz.	3	105
Veal			
arm steak			
lean	3 oz.	4	150
lean and fat	3 oz.	16	255
blade			
lean	3 oz.	7	200
lean and fat	3 oz.	14	240
cutlet			
breaded	3 oz.	13	270
round lean	3 oz.	11	170
round, lean and fat	3 oz.	13	240
loin medium fat, broiled	3 oz.	11	200
loin chop			
lean	3 oz.	5	150
lean and fat	3 oz.	11	215
rib chop			
lean	3 oz.	7	125
lean and fat	3 oz.	18	265
rump, marbled roasted	3 oz.	9	195
sirloin			
lean roasted	3 oz.	3	150
marbled roasted	3 oz.	6	155
sirloin steak, ground	3 oz.	14	230

Food Item	Amount	Fat Gm.	Calories
Meats (continued)			
Sirloin steak			
lean	3 oz.	5	175
lean and fat	3 oz.	17	260

Milk & Dairy Products

Food Item	Amount	Fat Gm.	Calories
Buttermilk			
1% fat	1 cup	2	100
dry	1 T.	0	25
Chocolate milk			
2% fat	1 cup	5	180
whole	1 cup	8	250
Condensed milk			
sweet	1/2 cup	14	440
sweet, fat-free	1/2 cup	0	440
Creamer, non dairy, Intl. vanilla	2 T.	3	80
Evaporated			
skim	1/2 cup	0	100
whole	1/2 cup	10	125
Half and half, fat-free	2 T.	0	20
Malted milk	1 cup	10	240
Milk			
non-fat dry powder	1/4 cup	0	110
skim fat	1 cup	0	90
1% fat	1 cup	3	100
2% fat	1 cup	5	120
Whole milk, 3.5% fat	1 cup	8	150
dry powder	1/4 cup	9	160
Milk shake			
chocolate	1 cup	17	340
soft serve	1 cup	7	220
vanilla	1 cup	15	270
Ovaltine w/ 1% milk	1 cup	3	170
Yogurt			
Dannon Lt/Crunchy car. apple	8 oz.	0	150
frozen, low fat	1/2 cup	3	115
frozen, non-fat	1/2 cup	0	80
fruit flavored, low fat	1 cup	3	225
fruit flavored, non-fat	1 cup	0	160
low fat	1 cup	3	145
plain	1 cup	8	190
skim, non-fat	1 cup	0	130
vanilla, low fat	1 cup	3	190
whole milk	1 cup	7	140
Yoplait Vanilla 'N Wafer	7 oz.	2	220

Miscellaneous

Food Item	Amount	Fat Gm.	Calories
Bac-Os	1 T.	1	30
Bouillon cube, beef or chicken	1	0	10
Chewing gum	1 stick	0	10
Gelatin, Jello	1/2 cup	0	80
Honey	1 T.	0	65
Horseradish	1 T.	1	12
Icing, decorator	1 T.	2	70
Icing, all varieties	1 T.	1	55
Jelly, all varieties	1 T.	0	50
Marmalade, citrus	1 T.	0	50
Meat tenderizer	1 tsp.	0	0
Molasses	1 T.	0	50
Olives			
black	2 large	4	40

Nutritional Information

Food Item	Amount	Fat Gm.	Calories
Miscellaneous (continued)			
Greek	3 medium	7	70
green	2 medium	2	15
Peanut butter			
regular	1 T.	9	150
Skippy reduced fat	1 T.	6	95
Pickle relish	1 T.	0	20
Pickles			
bread & butter	4 slices	0	20
dill	1 large	0	10
Kosher	1 oz.	0	10
sweet	1 oz.	0	145
Salt	1 tsp.	0	0
Shake 'n Bake, General Foods	1/4 pkg.	3	70
Spices and herbs	1 tsp.	0	5
Sugar substitutes	1 packet	0	5
Sugar, cane or beet	1 T.	0	45
Syrup, all varieties	1 T.	0	60
Vinegar	1 T.	0	0
Yeast	1 T.	0	20

Mixed Dishes

Food Item	Amount	Fat Gm.	Calories
Baked beans w/ pork	1 cup	4	270
Beans & franks, canned	1 cup	16	365
Beans, refried			
canned	1 cup	3	270
refried w/ fat	1 cup	26	540
refried, fat-free	1 cup	0	250
Beef & vegetable stew	1 cup	10	220
Beef burgundy	1 cup	21	330
Beef noodle casserole	1 cup	20	330
Beef Oriental, Lean Cuisine	1 serving	9	270
Beef pie, frozen	8 oz.	23	430
Beef stew	1 cup	8	180
Beef stew, homemade	1 cup	14	225
Beef teriyaki, Stouffer's	1 serving	11	365
Beef,			
chipped, creamed, homemade	1 cup	22	350
chipped, creamed, frozen	5 1/2 oz.	16	235
short ribs w/ gravy, frozen	6 oz.	28	380
sloppy joe	6 oz.	14	230
Burrito			
bean w/ cheese	1 large	10	230
bean w/o cheese	1 large	3	140
beef	1 large	25	425
with guacamole, frozen	6 oz.	16	350
Cabbage roll w/ beef & rice	1 average	8	170
Cannelloni, meat & cheese	1 piece	30	420
Cheese souffle	1 cup	11	175
Chicken			
à la king,			
Stouffer's	1 serving	11	330
Swanson's	1 serving	12	180
glazed, Lean Cuisine	1 serving	7	270
Chicken & dumplings	sm. serving	10	330
Chicken & noodles, Stouffer's	1 serving	15	250
Chicken & rice casserole	1 cup	18	365
Chicken & vegetable stir-fry	1 cup	7	140
Chicken Cacciatore, Stouffer's	1 serving	11	310
Chicken divan, Stouffer's	1 serving	22	335
Chicken-fried steak	4 oz.	25	400

Food Item	Amount	Fat Gm.	Calories
Mixed Dishes (continued)			
Chicken noodle casserole	1 cup	11	300
Chicken paprikash, Stouffer's	1 serving	15	390
Chicken pie			
frozen	8 oz.	23	400
homemade	8 oz.	32	550
Chicken salad, regular	4 oz.	21	280
Chili			
w/ beans	1 cup	15	300
w/o beans	1 cup	20	300
Chop suey			
beef	1 cup	17	300
chicken	1 cup	7	125
Chow mein			
beef, canned, La Choy	1 cup	2	70
chicken, canned, La Choy	1 cup	2	70
homemade	1 cup	9	220
Corned-beef hash	1 cup	23	375
Creamed chipped beef	1 cup	22	350
Deviled crab	1/2 cup	15	230
Deviled eggs	1/2 egg	5	70
Egg foo yung w/ sauce	1 piece	11	130
Egg salad	1/2 cup	17	210
Eggplant Parmesan	1 cup	24	350
Egg roll			
chicken, Chun King	1 average	7	210
homemade	1 average	10	150
pork, Chun King	1 average	8	220
Enchilada			
bean, beef, & cheese	1	14	250
beef, frozen	8 oz.	17	260
cheese, frozen	8 oz.	21	360
chicken, frozen	12 oz.	12	270
Fettuccine Alfredo	1 cup	30	460
Fillet of fish divan, frozen	8 oz.	2	180
Fish creole	1 cup	5	170
Fritter, corn	1 average	8	130
Frozen dinners			
chipped steak	18 oz.	40	730
chopped beefsteak	11 oz.	26	440
fried chicken	11 oz.	28	560
meat loaf	11 oz.	16	360
Salisbury steak	11 oz.	29	500
turkey	11 oz.	11	360
Green pepper stfd. w/ rice, beef	1 average	13	260
Ham salad w/ mayo	4 oz.	20	280
Ham spread, Spreadables	1/2 cup	19	205
Hamburger Helper, all types	8 oz.	19	375
Hamburger rice casserole	8 oz.	21	370
Lasagne			
cheese, frozen	8 oz.	11	320
homemade	1 serving	21	420
zucchini, Lean Cuisine	11 oz.	6	260
Lo mein, Chinese	1 cup	7	185
Lobster			
Cantonese	1 cup	20	335
Newburg	8 oz.	24	440
salad	1/2 cup	7	120
Macaroni & cheese			
box mix	1 cup	18	385
Kraft Thick 'n Creamy	2/3 cup	5	510

Nutritional Information

Food Item	Amount	Fat Gm.	Calories
Mixed Dishes (continued)			
Macaroni & cheese, frozen	6 oz.	12	260
Manicotti, cheese & tomato	1 piece	11	240
Meat loaf, w/ reg. ground beef	3 oz.	18	280
Onion rings	10 average	17	230
Oysters Rockefeller	6-8 oysters	14	230
Pizza			
cheese	1 slice	10	180
cheese, French bread, frozen	5 1/8 oz.	13	330
combination w/ meat	1 slice	17	270
deep dish, cheese	1 slice	13	420
pepperoni, frozen	1 slice	18	360
Pizza rolls, Jeno's	3 pieces	7	130
Pork, sweet & sour	1 1/2 cup	22	390
Quiche			
Lorraine (bacon)	1 slice	20	360
plain or vegetable	1 slice	17	310
Ratatouille	1/2 cup	7	90
Ravioli, canned	1 cup	7	240
Ravioli w/ meat & tomato sauce	1 piece	3	50
Salisbury steak w/ gravy	8 oz.	27	365
Salmon patty, homemade	6 oz.	20	400
Sandwiches			
BLT w/ mayo	1	16	280
chicken w/ mayo	1	14	300
club house w/ mayo	1	20	590
corned beef on rye	1	11	290
egg salad	1	12	280
ham & mayo	1	10	280
peanut butter & jelly	1	10	370
Reuben	1	33	530
roast beef & gravy	1	25	430
roast beef & mayo	1	22	430
sub w/ salami & cheese	1	41	780
tuna salad	1	14	280
turkey, lettuce, & mayo	1	18	400
turkey breast	1	5	285
Shepherd's pie	12 oz.	24	400
Shrimp creole	1 cup	20	150
Spaghetti			
w/ meat sauce	1 cup	16	320
w/ tomato sauce	1 cup	2	180
Spaghetti Os, Franco American	1 cup	2	160
Spinach souffle	1 cup	15	210
Stroganoff, beef, Stouffer's	9 3/4 oz.	20	390
Sweet & sour pork	1 cup	22	380
Taco beef	1 medium	17	270
Tortellini, meat or cheese	1 cup	15	360
Tostada w/ refried beans	1 medium	16	290
Tuna Helper	1 cup	10	295
Tuna noodle casserole	1 cup	13	315
Tuna salad			
oil pack w/ mayo	1/2 cup	16	220
water pack w/ mayo	1/2 cup	10	170
Veal Parmigiana			
frozen	6 oz.	20	340
homemade	1 cup	25	485
scallopini	1 cup	20	420
Welsh rarebit	1 cup	30	415
Won Ton w/ pork, fried	1 piece	4	80
Yorkshire pudding	1 serving	3	50

Food Item	Amount	Fat Gm.	Calories
Nuts & Seeds			
Almonds	12-15	9	105
Brazil nuts	4 medium	11	115
Cashews, roasted	6-8	8	95
Chestnuts, fresh	3 small	1	65
Coconut, dried, shredded	1/3 cup	9	135
Hazelnuts (filberts)	10-12	11	105
Macadamia nuts, roasted	6 medium	12	120
Mixed nuts			
dry roasted	1 oz.	14	160
w/ peanuts	1 oz.	15	150
w/o peanuts	1 oz.	16	175
Peanut butter			
creamy or chunky	1 T.	8	90
Skippy reduced fat	1 T.	6	95
Peanuts			
chopped	2 T.	9	100
honey roasted	2 T.	9	110
in shell	1 cup	18	210
Pecans	2 T.	9	90
Pine nuts (pignolia)	2 T.	9	85
Pistachios	2 T.	8	90
Poppy seeds	1 T.	4	45
Sesame nut mix	2 T.	5	65
Sesame seeds	2 T.	9	95
Sunflower seeds	2 T.	9	100
Trail mix w/ seeds, nuts			
carob	2 T.	5	85
walnut	2 T.	8	80
Pasta & Rice			
Macaroni			
semolina or durham	1 cup	1	160
whole wheat	1 cup	1	180
Noodles			
Alfredo	1 cup	30	460
almondine, from mix	1/4 pkg.	12	240
cellophane, fried	1 cup	4	140
egg	1 cup	2	200
mostaccioli	1 cup	2	200
ramen, all varieties	1 cup	6	190
rice	1 cup	0	140
Romanoff	1 cup	23	370
Red beans and rice, Vigo	1/3 cup	0	190
Rice			
brown	1/2 cup	1	115
fried	1/2 cup	7	180
long grain, wild	1/2 cup	2	120
pilaf	1/2 cup	7	170
Spanish style	1/2 cup	2	105
white	1/2 cup	1	110
Rice A Roni	1/2 cup	1	110
Spaghetti, enriched	1 cup	1	160
Poultry			
Chicken			
Breast			
w/ skin, fried	1/2 breast	10	235
w/o skin, fried	1/2 breast	6	180
w/ skin, roasted	1/2 breast	8	190

Nutritional Information

Poultry (continued)

Food Item	Amount	Fat Gm.	Calories
w/o skin, roasted	1/2 breast	3	140
Fryers			
w/ skin, batter dipped, fried	3 oz.	15	250
w/o skin, fried	3 oz.	9	205
w/ skin, roasted	3 oz.	12	205
w/o skin roasted	3 oz.	6	160
Leg			
w/ skin, fried	1 leg	8	120
w/ skin, roasted	1 leg	6	110
w/o skin roasted	1 leg	2	75
Roll, light meat	3 oz.	6	135
Thigh			
w/ skin, fried	1 thigh	12	180
w/ skin, roasted	1 thigh	10	150
w/o skin, roasted	1 thigh	6	110
Wing			
w/ skin, fried	1 wing	9	120
w/ skin, roasted	1 wing	7	100
w/o skin, roasted	1 wing	3	70
Duck			
w/ skin, roasted	3 oz.	24	290
w/o skin, roasted	3 oz.	10	175
Pheasant, raw breast	3 oz.	3	120
Turkey			
white meat,			
oven roasted	3 oz.	3	100
smoked	3 oz.	4	105
dark meat			
w/ skin, roasted	3 oz.	10	190
w/o skin, roasted	3 oz.	6	160
ground, mixed meat	3 oz.	12	195
ground, all white meat	3 oz.	4	110
ham, cured	3 oz.	4	110
light meat			
w/ skin, roasted	3 oz.	7	170
w/o skin, roasted	3 oz.	3	135
loaf, breast meat	3 oz.	2	95
pastrami	1 oz.	1	40
patties, breaded, fried	1 patty	17	265
roll, light meat	3 oz.	6	125
salami	1 oz.	4	55
sausage, cooked	1 oz.	3	50
sliced w/ gravy, frozen	5 oz.	4	95

Salads

Food Item	Amount	Fat Gm.	Calories
Caesar salad w/o anchovies	1 cup	9	80
Carrot-raisin salad	1/2 cup	8	315
Chef salad w/o dressing	1 cup	8	110
Coleslaw			
w/ mayo-type dressing	1/2 cup	14	145
w/ vinaigrette	1/2 cup	5	75
Fruit salad			
fresh	1/2 cup	0	70
w/ mayo dressing	1/2 cup	8	220
Gelatin salad w/ fruit	1/2 cup	0	20
Macaroni salad w/ mayo	1/2 cup	13	200
Pasta primavera salad	1/2 cup	10	200
Potato salad	1 cup	20	360
German style	1/2 cup	3	140
w/ mayo dressing	1/2 cup	11	190

Salads (continued)

Food Item	Amount	Fat Gm.	Calories
Seven-layer salad	1 cup	18	225
Taco salad w/ taco sauce	1 cup	14	200
Three-bean salad	1/2 cup	11	145
Three-bean salad, no oil	1/2 cup	0	90
Tuna salad, w/ mayo	1/2 cup	19	285
Waldorf salad w/ mayo	1/2 cup	25	310

Salad Dressings

Food Item	Amount	Fat Gm.	Calories
Blue Cheese			
fat-free	1 oz.	0	20
regular	1 oz.	16	155
Buttermilk, from mix	1 oz.	12	120
Caesar	1 oz.	14	140
French			
creamy	1 oz.	14	140
reduced fat	1 oz.	2	40
regular	1 oz.	13	140
Green Goddess			
reduced fat	1 oz.	4	60
regular	1 oz.	14	140
Honey mustard	1 oz.	13	180
Italian			
creamy	1 oz.	9	100
reduced fat	1 oz.	3	30
regular zesty from mix	1 oz.	18	170
Kraft free	1 oz.	0	40
Kraft reduced calorie	1 oz.	2	50
Mayonnaise type			
reduced fat	1 oz.	4	40
regular	1 oz.	10	120
Oil & vinegar	1 oz.	15	140
Ranch			
w/ mayo	1 oz.	16	160
reduced fat	1 oz.	10	110
Russian			
reduced fat	1 oz.	1	45
regular	1 oz.	16	150
Sesame seed	1 oz.	14	140
Sweet & sour	1 oz.	2	60
Thousand Island			
reduced fat	1 oz.	3	50
regular	1 oz.	11	60

Snack Foods

Food Item	Amount	Fat Gm.	Calories
Bagel chips or crisps	1 oz.	9	150
Bugles	1 oz.	8	150
Bugles Lite	1 oz.	2	85
Cheese Puff Balls, Cheetos	1 oz.	11	160
Cheese Puffs, Cheetos	1 oz.	10	160
Cheese Balls, Planter's red. fat	30	3	70
Chex Mix, traditional	1 cup	5	195
Corn chips, Frito's			
lite	1 oz.	10	145
regular	1 oz.	10	155
Corn nuts, all flavors	1 oz.	4	120
Cracker Jacks	1 oz.	1	115
Doo-Dads, Nabisco	1/2 cup	6	140
Handisnacks, Cheez'n Pretzel	1 serving	6	110
Party mix (cereal, pretzels, nuts)	1 cup	23	310
Popcorn, air popped	1 cup	0	20

Nutritional Information

Food Item	Amount	Fat Gm.	Calories
Snack Foods (continued)			
Popcorn (continued)			
Betty Crocker 94% fat-free	3 cups	1	55
caramel	1 cup	4	140
Cracker Jack, fat-free	1 cup	0	110
Healthy Choice	3 cups	1	60
microwave, plain	1 cup	3	50
microwave, w/ butter	1 cup	4	60
popped w/ oil	1 cup	2	40
Potato chips			
individually	10 chips	8	110
by weight	1 oz.	11	160
barbecue flavor	1 oz.	9	150
lite, Pringles	1 oz.	8	145
regular, Pringles	1 oz.	13	170
Potato Crisps, Frito Lay, baked	16	2	135
Potato sticks	1 oz.	10	150
Pretzels			
hard	1 oz.	1	110
soft	1 average	0	175
Rice cakes, Quaker caramel	1 cake	1	50
Tortilla chips			
baked w/o oil	1 oz.	1	100
Doritos	1 oz.	7	140
Tostitos	1 oz.	8	145

Soups

Food Item	Amount	Fat Gm.	Calories
Asparagus			
cream of, w/ milk	1 cup	8	160
cream of, w/ water	1 cup	4	90
Bean			
w/ bacon	1 cup	6	175
w/ franks	1 cup	7	190
w/ ham	1 cup	8	230
w/o meat	1 cup	3	140
Beef			
broth	1 cup	0	30
chunky	1 cup	5	170
Beef barley	1 cup	1	70
Beef noodle	1 cup	3	85
Broccoli, creamy w/ water	1 cup	3	70
Campbell's Chunky			
w/ meat	1 cup	5	170
w/o meat	1 cup	4	120
Canned vegetable type w/o meat	1 cup	2	70
Cheese w/ milk	1 cup	15	230
Chicken			
chunky	1 cup	7	180
cream of, w/ milk	1 cup	11	190
cream of, w/ water	1 cup	7	115
Chicken and dumplings	1 cup	5	100
Chicken/beef noodle or vegetable	1 cup	3	80
Chicken gumbo	1 cup	1	55
Chicken mushroom	1 cup	9	150
Chicken noodle			
chunky	1 cup	6	115
w/ water	1 cup	2	75
Chicken vegetable			
chunky	1 cup	5	165
w/ water	1 cup	3	75
Chicken w/ noodles, chunky	1 cup	5	180

Food Item	Amount	Fat Gm.	Calories
Soups (continued)			
Chicken w/ rice			
chunky	1 cup	3	125
w/ water	1 cup	2	60
Chicken wild rice	1 cup	2	75
Clam chowder			
Manhattan chunky	1 cup	3	135
New England	1 cup	7	160
Consomme w/ gelatin	1 cup	0	30
Crab	1 cup	1	80
Dehydrated soups			
asparagus, cream of	1 cup	2	60
bean w/ bacon	1 cup	3	105
beef broth cube	1 cup	0	10
beef noodle	1 cup	1	40
cauliflower	1 cup	2	70
chicken, cream of	1 cup	5	110
chicken broth cube	1 cup	0	10
chicken noodle	1 cup	1	50
chicken rice	1 cup	1	60
clam chowder			
Manhattan	1 cup	2	65
New England	1 cup	4	95
minestrone	1 cup	2	80
mushroom	1 cup	5	95
onion	1 package	2	115
tomato	1 cup	2	100
vegetable beef	1 cup	1	50
Gazpacho	1 cup	0	40
Healthy Request			
cream of mushroom	1 cup	3	70
cream of chicken	1 cup	3	80
Homemade or restaurant style			
beer cheese	1 cup	23	310
cauliflower, cream of, whl mlk	1 cup	10	165
celery, cream of, whole milk	1 cup	11	165
chicken broth	1 cup	1	40
clam chowder			
Manhattan	1 cup	2	80
New England	1 cup	14	270
corn chowder	1 cup	12	250
fish chowder w/ whole milk	1 cup	13	285
Gazpacho	1 cup	7	100
Mock turtle	1 cup	15	245
Onion, French w/o cheese	1 cup	6	90
Oyster stew w/ whole milk	1 cup	17	270
Seafood gumbo	1 cup	4	155
Lentil	1 cup	1	160
Minestrone			
chunky	1 cup	3	130
w/ water	1 cup	2	80
Mushroom, cream of			
condensed	1 cup	23	310
w/ milk	1 cup	14	200
w/ water	1 cup	9	130
reduced fat	1 cup	7	140
Onion	1 cup	2	60
Oyster stew w/ water	1 cup	4	60
Pea			
green, w/ water	1 cup	3	165
split	1 cup	1	60

Nutritional Information

Food Item	Amount	Fat Gm.	Calories
Soups (continued)			
split w/ ham	1 cup	4	190
Potato, cream of, w/ milk	1 cup	7	160
Shrimp, cream of, w/ milk	1 cup	9	165
Tomato			
w/ milk	1 cup	6	160
w/ water	1 cup	2	100
Tomato bisque w/ milk	1 cup	7	100
Tomato rice	1 cup	3	120
Turkey, chunky	1 cup	4	135
Turkey noodle	1 cup	2	70
Turkey vegetable	1 cup	3	75
Vegetable, chunky	1 cup	4	120
Vegetable w/ beef, chunky	1 cup	3	135
Vegetable w/ beef, broth	1 cup	2	80
Vegetarian vegetable	1 cup	2	70
Won Ton	1 cup	2	90

Spreads, Oils & Creams

Food Item	Amount	Fat Gm.	Calories
Butter			
solid	1 T.	12	110
whipped	1 T.	9	90
Butter Buds, liquid	2 T.	0	10
Cream			
light	1 T.	3	30
medium (25% fat)	1 T.	4	40
Cream substitute			
liquid/frozen	1/2 fl. oz.	1	20
powdered	1 T.	1	10
Dijonnaise	1 T.	3	30
Half & Half	1 T.	2	20
Margarine			
liquid	1 T.	11	100
solid (corn)	1 T.	10	90
Mayonnaise			
low fat	1 T.	1	25
regular	1 T.	11	100
Miracle Whip	1	7	70
Mustard	1 T.	1	10
No-stick spray, fat-free, all types	1 spray	1	50
Oil			
canola	1 T.	14	120
corn	1 T.	14	120
olive	1 T.	14	120
safflower	1 T.	14	120
soybean	1 T.	14	120
Sandwich spread, non-fat	1 T	0	25
Shortening, vegetable	1 T.	12	105
Sour cream			
cultured	1 T.	2	25
half & half, cultured	1 T.	2	20
imitation	1 T.	3	25
reduced calorie	1 T.	1	15
fat-free	1 T.	0	45
Tartar sauce	1 T.	8	75

Vegetables

Food Item	Amount	Fat Gm.	Calories
Alfalfa sprouts, raw	1 cup	0	5
Artichoke, boiled	1 medium	0	50
Artichoke hearts, boiled	1/2 cup	0	40
Asparagus, cooked	1/2 cup	0	20

Food Item	Amount	Fat Gm.	Calories
Vegetables (continued)			
Avocado	1 average	28	325
Bamboo shoots, raw	1/2 cup	0	20
Beans, baked			
all types cooked w/o fat	1/2 cup	0	125
baked, brown sugar & molasses	1/2 cup	1	130
baked, Bush's vegetarian	1/2 cup	0	130
baked w/ pork & tomato sauce	1/2 cup	2	190
baked, vegetarian	1/2 cup	1	160
homestyle canned	1/2 cup	2	130
refried			
Old El Paso fat-free	1/2 cup	0	110
Ortego 98% fat-free	1/2 cup	3	140
Beets	1/2 cup	0	35
Black-eyed peas, cooked	1/2 cup	0	100
Broccoli			
cooked	1/2 cup	0	45
frozen in butter sauce	1/2 cup	2	50
frozen w/ cheese sauce	1/2 cup	6	115
frozen, chopped, cooked	1/2 cup	0	25
raw	1/2 cup	0	10
Brussels sprouts, cooked	1/2 cup	0	30
Butter beans, canned	1/2 cup	1	100
Cabbage			
Chinese, raw	1 cup	0	10
green cooked	1/2 cup	0	15
red, raw, shredded	1/2 cup	0	10
Carrot			
cooked	1/2 cup	0	35
raw	1/2 cup	0	30
Cauliflower			
cooked	1/2 cup	0	15
frozen w/ cheese sauce	1/2 cup	6	115
raw	1/2 cup	0	10
Celery			
cooked	1/2 cup	0	10
raw	1 stalk	0	5
Chard, cooked	1/2 cup	0	20
Chilies, green	1/4 cup	0	15
Chinese-style vegetables, frozen	1/2 cup	5	80
Collard greens, cooked	1/2 cup	0	15
Corn			
corn on the cob	1 medium	1	80
cream style, canned	1/2 cup	0	95
frozen, cooked	1/2 cup	0	65
frozen w/ butter sauce	1/2 cup	3	105
whole kernel, cooked	1/2 cup	1	90
Cucumber			
w/ skin	1/2 medium	0	10
w/o skin	1/2 cup	0	5
Eggplant, cooked	1/2 cup	0	15
Endive lettuce	1 cup	0	10
Garbanzo beans	1/2 cup	2	135
Green beans			
French style, cooked	1/2 cup	0	20
snap, cooked	1/2 cup	0	20
Hominy, white or yellow, cooked	1 cup	1	140
Italian-style vegetables, frozen	1/2 cup	7	130
Kidney beans	1/2 cup	0	110
Leeks, chopped, raw	1/2 cup	0	35
Lentils, cooked	1/2 cup	0	115

Nutritional Information

Food Item	Amount	Fat Gm.	Calories
Vegetables (continued)			
Lettuce, leaf	1/2 cup	0	5
Lima beans, cooked	1/2 cup	0	110
Mushrooms			
canned	1/2 cup	0	20
fried sauteed	5 medium	10	100
raw	1/2 cup	0	10
Mustard greens, cooked	1/2 cup	0	15
Okra, cooked	1/2 cup	0	25
Onions			
canned, french fried	1 oz.	15	175
chopped, raw	1/2 cup	0	25
Parsley, chopped, raw	1/2 cup	0	10
Parsnips, cooked	1/2 cup	0	65
Peas, green, cooked	1/2 cup	0	70
Pepper, bell, chopped, raw	1/2 cup	0	10
Pimientos, canned	3 oz.	0	30
Potato			
au gratin			
from mix	1/2 cup	6	140
homemade	1/2 cup	9	160
baked w/ skin	1 medium	0	220
boiled w/o skin	1/2 cup	0	115
French fries			
frozen, baked	10 pieces	4	110
homemade, fried	10 pieces	8	160
hash browns	1/2 cup	11	165
knishes	1	3	75
mashed			
from flakes	1/2 cup	0	80
w/ milk & margarine	1/2 cup	4	110
pan fried, O'Brien	1/2 cup	2	80
scalloped			
from mix	1/2 cup	6	125
homemade	1/2 cup	5	105
w/ cheese	1/2 cup	10	175
potato pancakes	8" cake	13	400
potato puffs, frozen	1 puff	1	15
twice-baked potato w/ cheese	1 medium	10	180
Pumpkin, canned	1/2 cup	0	40
Radish, raw	10	0	5
Rhubarb, raw	1 cup	0	30
Sauerkraut, canned	1/2 cup	0	20
Scallions, raw	5 medium	0	45
Soybeans, mature, cooked	1/2 cup	8	150
Spinach			
cooked	1/2 cup	0	20
creamed	1/2 cup	6	90
raw	1 cup	0	10
Squash			
acorn, baked	1/2 cup	0	55
butternut, cooked	1/2 cup	0	40
summer			
cooked	1/2 cup	0	20
raw, sliced	1/2 cup	0	15
winter, cooked	1/2 cup	0	40
Sweet potato			
baked	1 medium	0	120
candied	1/2 cup	4	190
mashed w/o fat	1/2 cup	0	170
Tofu, raw	4 oz.	5	85

Food Item	Amount	Fat Gm.	Calories
Vegetables (continued)			
Tomato			
raw	1 medium	0	25
stewed	1/2 cup	0	35
tomato paste, canned	1/2 cup	1	110
tomato sauce, plain	1/2 cup	0	30
Turnips, cooked	1/2 cup	0	15
Water chestnuts, canned, sliced	1/2 cup	0	35
Watercress, raw	1/2 cup	0	0
Wax beans, canned	1/2 cup	0	25
Yams, baked	1/2 cup	0	80
Zucchini, cooked	1/2 cup	0	15

Note: Nutritional values vary between different brands. The values shown in this book represent an average. Fat gram values have been rounded off to the nearest whole number and calories have been rounded off to the nearest 5.

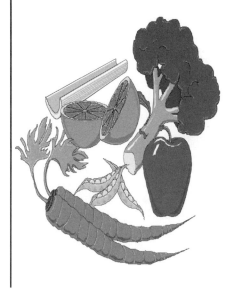

Fast Food Nutritional Information

Food Item	Amount	Fat Gm.	Calories
Arby's®			
Breakfast Items			
Bacon	1 serving	7	90
Biscuit (Plain)	1	15	280
Blueberry Muffin	1	9	230
Cinnamon Nut Danish	1	11	360
Croissant (Plain)	1	12	220
Egg Portion	1 serving	8	95
French-Toastix	1 serving	21	430
Ham	1 serving	1	45
Sausage	1 serving	15	165
Swiss	1 serving	3	45
Table Syrup	1 serving	0	100
Roast Beef Sandwiches			
Arby's Melt with cheddar	1	18	370
Arby-Q	1	18	430
Bac'n Cheddar Deluxe	1	34	540
Beef'n Cheddar	1	28	485
Giant Roast Beef	1	28	555
Junior Roast Beef	1	14	320
Regular Roast Beef	1	19	390
Super Roast Beef	1	27	520
Chicken			
Breaded Chicken Fillet	1	28	535
Chicken Cordon Bleu	1	33	620
Chicken Fingers (2 pieces)	1	16	290
Grilled Chicken BBQ	1	13	390
Grilled Chicken Deluxe	1	20	430
Roast Chicken Club	1	31	545
Roast Chicken Deluxe	1	22	430
Roast Chicken Santa Fe	1	22	435
Sub Roll Sandwiches			
French Dip	1	22	475
Hot Ham 'n Swiss	1	23	500
Italian Sub	1	36	675
Philly Beef 'n Swiss	1	47	755
Roast Beef Sub	1	42	700
Triple Cheese Melt	1	45	720
Turkey Sub	1	27	550
Light Menu			
Roast Beef Deluxe	1	10	295
Roast Chicken Deluxe	1	6	275
Roast Turkey Deluxe	1	7	260
Garden Salad	1	1	60
Roast Chicken Salad	1	2	150
Side Salad	1	1	25
Other Sandwiches			
Fish Fillet	1	27	530
Ham 'n Cheese	1	14	360
Ham 'n Cheese Melt	1	13	330
Potatoes			
Cheddar Curly Fries	1 serving	18	330
Curly Fries	1 serving	15	300
French Fries	1 serving	13	245

Food Item	Amount	Fat Gm.	Calories
Potatoes (continued)			
Potato Cakes	1 serving	12	205
Baked Potato (plain)	1	1	355
Baked Potato w/ marg. & sour cm.	1	24	580
Broccoli 'n Cheddar Baked Potato	1	20	570
Deluxe Baked Potato	1	36	735
Soups			
Boston Clam Chowder	1 serving	9	190
Cream of Broccoli	1 serving	8	160
Lumberjack Mixed Vegetable	1 serving	4	90
Old Fashion Chicken Noodle	1 serving	2	80
Potato with Bacon	1 serving	7	170
Timberline Chili	1 serving	10	220
Wisconsin Cheese	1 serving	18	280
Desserts			
Apple Turnover	1	14	330
Cherry Turnover	1	13	320
Cheesecake (plain)	1	23	320
Chocolate Chip Cookie	1 serving	6	125
Chocolate Shake	1	12	450
Jomocha Shake	1	10	385
Vanilla Shake	1	12	360
Butterfinger Polar Swirl	1	18	455
Heath Polar Swirl	1	22	540
Oreo Polar Swirl	1	22	480
Peanut Butter Cup Polar Swirl	1	24	515
Snickers Polar Swirl	1	19	510
Sauces			
Arby's Sauce	1/2 oz.	1	15
Horsey Sauce	1/2 oz.	5	60
Boston Market®			
Entrees			
Chicken			
white meat, no skin or wing	1/4 chicken	4	160
white meat w/ skin	1/4 chicken	17	330
dark meat, no skin	1/4 chicken	10	210
dark meat w/ skin	1/4 chicken	22	330
1/2 chicken w/ skin	1/2 chicken	37	630
chicken pot pie	1 pie	34	750
chicken salad	3/4 cup	30	390
Turkey breast, skinless, rotisserie	5 oz.	1	170
Ham w/ cinnamon apples	8 oz.	13	350
Meat loaf & chunky tomato sauce	8 oz.	18	370
Meat loaf & brown gravy	7 oz.	22	390
Soups, Salads, Sandwiches			
Caesar salad entree	10 oz.	43	520
w/o dressing	8 oz.	13	240
Chicken caesar salad	13 oz.	47	670
Chicken sandwich/cheese sauce	1	32	760
w/o cheese sauce	1	4	430
Chicken salad sandwich	1	33	680
Chicken soup	3/4 cup	3	80
Chicken tortilla soup	1 cup	11	220
Turkey sandwich/cheese sauce	1	28	710
without cheese sauce	1	4	400

Fast Food Nutritional Information

Food Item	Amount	Fat Gm.	Calories
Boston Market (continued)			
Ham sandwich w/ cheese sauce	1	35	760
w/o cheese sauce	1	9	450
Ham & turkey club w/ ch. & sc.	1	43	890
w/o cheese or sauce	1	6	430
Meat loaf sandwich w/ cheese	1	33	860
w/o cheese	1	21	690
Hot Side Dishes			
Steamed vegetables	2/3 cup	1	35
New potatoes	3/4 cup	3	140
Buttered corn	3/4 cup	4	190
Zucchini marinara	3/4 cup	4	80
Mashed potatoes	2/3 cup	8	180
w/ gravy	3/4 cup	9	200
Chicken gravy	1 oz.	1	15
Rice pilaf	2/3 cup	5	180
Creamed spinach	3/4 cup	24	300
Stuffing	3/4 cup	12	310
Butternut squash	3/4 cup	6	160
Macaroni & cheese	3/4 cup	10	280
BBQ baked beans	3/4 cup	9	330
Cinnamon apples	3/4 cup	5	250
Cold Side Dishes			
Fruit salad	3/4 cup	1	70
Mediterranean pasta salad	3/4 cup	10	170
Cranberry relish	3/4 cup	5	370
Cole slaw	3/4 cup	16	280
Tortellini salad	3/4 cup	24	380
Caesar side salad	4 oz.	17	210
Baked Goods			
Brownie	1	27	450
Corn bread	1 loaf	6	200
Oatmeal raisin cookie	1	13	320
Chocolate chip cookie	1	17	340

Burger King®

Food Item	Amount	Fat Gm.	Calories
Breakfast			
Croissan'wich w/ bcn., egg/ chs.	1	24	350
Croissan'wich w/ sg., egg & chs.	1	41	530
Croissan'wich w/ ham, egg/chs.	1	22	350
French Toast Sticks	1 serving	27	500
Hash Browns	1 serving	12	220
A.M. Express Jam			
grape	1 pkg.	0	30
strawberry	1 pkg.	0	30
Burgers			
Whopper	1	39	640
Whopper w/ cheese	1	46	730
Double Whopper	1	56	870
Double Whopper w/ cheese	1	63	960
Whopper Jr.	1	24	420
Whopper Jr. w/ cheese	1	28	460
Hamburger	1	15	330
Cheeseburger	1	19	380
Double Cheeseburger	1	36	600
Double Cheeseburger w/ bacon	1	39	640

Food Item	Amount	Fat Gm.	Calories
Sandwich/Side Orders			
BK Big Fish Sandwich	1	43	720
Bk Broiler Chicken Sandwich	1	29	540
Chicken Sandwich	1	43	700
Chicken Tenders	6 pieces	12	250
Broiled Chicken Salad w/o drsg.	1	10	200
Garden Salad w/o dressing	1	5	90
Side Salad	1	3	50
French Fries (medium)	1 serving	20	400
Onion Rings	1	14	310
Dutch Apple Pie	1	15	310

Dairy Queen®

Food Item	Amount	Fat Gm.	Calories
DQ Brazier Entrees			
Single Hamburger	1	13	310
Single hamburger w/ cheese	1	18	365
Double hamburger	1	25	460
Double hamburger w/ cheese	1	34	570
DQ Homestyle® Ultimate burger	1	47	700
Hot dog	1	16	280
Hot dog w/ cheese	1	21	330
Hot dog w/ chili	1	19	320
1/4 pound Super Dog™	1	38	590
BBQ beef sandwich	1	4	225
Grilled chicken fillet sandwich	1	8	300
Breaded chicken fillet sandwich	1	20	430
w/ cheese	1	25	480
Fish fillet sandwich	1	16	370
w/ cheese	1	21	420
Salads & Sides			
Side salad without dressing	1 serving	0	25
Garden salad	1 serving	13	200
Thousand Island dressing	2 oz.	21	225
Reduced calorie French dressing	2 oz.	5	90
French fries			
small	1 serving	10	210
medium	1 serving	14	300
large	1 serving	18	390
Onion rings	1 serving	12	240
Desserts			
Vanilla cone			
small	1 serving	4	140
regular	1 serving	7	230
large	1 serving	10	340
Chocolate cone			
regular	1 serving	7	230
large	1 serving	11	350
Chocolate dipped cone, regular	1 serving	16	330
Chocolate sundae, regular	1 serving	7	300
Vanilla shake			
regular	1 serving	14	520
large	1 serving	16	600
Chocolate shake, regular	1 serving	14	540
Vanilla Malt, regular	1 serving	14	610
Banana split	1 serving	11	510
Peanut Buster® Parfait	1 serving	32	710
Hot Fudge Brownie Delight®	1 serving	29	710
Nutty Double Fudge™	1 serving	22	580

Fast Food Nutritional Information

Food Item	Amount	Fat Gm.	Calories
Dairy Queen® (continued)			
Strawberry Blizzard®			
small	1 serving	12	400
regular	1 serving	16	570
Small Heath Blizzard®	1 serving	23	560
Heath Blizzard®, regular	1 serving	36	820
Strbry. Waffle Cone Sundae™	1 serving	12	350
Buster Bar®	1 serving	29	450
Dilly® Bar	1 serving	13	210
DQ® Sandwich	1 serving	4	140
DQ® Frozen Cake Slice	1 serving	18	380
Mr. Misty®, regular	1 serving	0	250
Yogurt Cone			
regular	1 serving	1	180
large	1 serving	1	260
Cup of yogurt			
regular	1 serving	1	170
large	1 serving	1	230
Yogurt strawberry sundae, reg.	1 serving	1	200
Strawberry Breeze®			
regular	1 serving	1	420
small	1 serving	1	290
Heath Breeze®			
regular	1 serving	21	680
small	1 serving	12	450
DQ Big Scoop®			
chocolate	1 serving	14	310
vanilla	1 serving	14	300

Domino's® Pizza

12" Thin Crust

Food Item	Amount	Fat Gm.	Calories
Cheese	1/3 pizza	16	365
Pepperoni	1/3 pizza	23	450
Extra cheese & pepperoni	1/3 pizza	28	510
Ham	1/3 pizza	17	390
Italian sausage & mushroom	1/3 pizza	21	440
Veggie	1/3 pizza	17	385

12" Deep Dish

Food Item	Amount	Fat Gm.	Calories
Cheese	1/4 pie	24	560
Pepperoni	1/4 pie	29	620
Extra cheese & pepperoni	1/4 pie	33	670
Ham	1/4 pie	25	575
Italian sausage & mushroom	1/4 pie	28	620
Veggie	1/4 pie	25	575

12" Hand Tossed

Food Item	Amount	Fat Gm.	Calories
Cheese	1/4 pie	10	345
Pepperoni	1/4 pie	15	405
Extra Cheese & Pepperoni	1/4 pie	19	455
Ham	1/4 pie	10	360
Italian sausage & mushroom	1/4 pie	14	400
Veggie	1/4 pie	10	360

Kentucky Fried Chicken®

Chicken Entrees

Food Item	Amount	Fat Gm.	Calories
Colonel's Rotisserie Gold®			
Chicken Quarter			
breast & wing	1 serving	19	335
w/ skin removed	1 serving	6	200

Food Item	Amount	Fat Gm.	Calories
KFC® (continued)			
leg & thigh	1 serving	24	335
w/ skin removed	1 serving	12	215
Original Recipe® Chicken			
whole wing	1 serving	8	150
breast	1 serving	20	360
drumstick	1 serving	7	130
thigh	1 serving	17	260
Extra Tasty Crispy™ Chicken			
whole wing	1 serving	13	200
breast	1 serving	28	470
drumstick	1 serving	11	190
thigh	1 serving	25	370
Hot & Spicy Chicken			
whole wing	1 serving	15	210
breast	1 serving	35	530
drumstick	1 serving	11	190
thigh	1 serving	27	370

Snackables

Food Item	Amount	Fat Gm.	Calories
Hot Wings™	6 pieces	33	470
Colonel's™ Chicken Sandwich	1 serving	27	480
Value BBQ Fl. Chicken Sandwich	1 serving	8	255
Kentucky Nuggets®	6 nuggets	18	285
Chicken pot pie	1 serving	35	700
Crispy Strips	1 serving	19	320

Sides & Salads

Food Item	Amount	Fat Gm.	Calories
Corn-on-the-cob	1 serving	12	220
Green beans	1 serving	1	35
BBQ baked beans	1 serving	2	130
Macaroni & cheese	1 serving	8	160
Mean Greens™	1 serving	2	50
Red beans & rice	1 serving	3	115
Biscuit	1 biscuit	12	200
Corn bread	1 serving	13	230
Cole slaw	1 serving	6	115
Potato salad	1 serving	11	180
Mashed potatoes w/ gravy	1 serving	5	110
Potato wedges	1 serving	9	190
Garden rice	1 serving	1	75

McDonald's®

Breakfast

Food Item	Amount	Fat Gm.	Calories
Egg McMuffin®	1 serving	13	290
Sausage McMuffin®	1 serving	23	360
Sausage McMuffin® with egg	1 serving	29	440
English muffin	1 serving	2	140
Sausage biscuit	1 serving	29	430
Sausage biscuit with egg	1 serving	35	520
Bacon, egg & cheese biscuit	1 serving	26	440
Biscuit	1	13	260
Sausage	1 serving	16	170
Scrambled eggs	2	12	170
Hash browns	1 serving	8	130
Hotcakes, plain	1 serving	7	310
Hotcakes w/ 2 pats marg. & syrup	1 serving	16	580
Breakfast Burrito	1	20	320
Fat-free apple bran muffin	1 serving	0	170
Apple danish	1 serving	16	360

Fast Food Nutritional Information

Food Item	Amount	Fat Gm.	Calories
McDonalds® Entrees (continued)			
Cinnamon roll	1 roll	20	400
Cheese danish	1 serving	22	410
Cinnamon raisin danish	1 serving	22	430
Raspberry danish	1 serving	16	400
Entrees			
Hamburger	1 serving	10	270
Cheeseburger	1 serving	14	320
Quarter Pounder®	1 serving	21	430
Quarter Pounder® w/ cheese	1 serving	30	530
Big Mac®	1 serving	28	530
Arch Deluxe™	1 serving	31	570
Arch Deluxe™ with bacon	1 serving	34	610
Filet-O-Fish®	1 serving	16	360
Fish Fillet Deluxe™	1 serving	20	510
McGrilled Chicken Classic®	1 serving	4	260
McChicken® Sandwich	1 serving	30	510
Grilled Chicken Deluxe	1 serving	6	330
Crispy Chicken Deluxe	1 serving	26	530
Chicken McNuggets			
4 pieces	1 serving	11	190
6 pieces	1 serving	17	290
9 pieces	1 serving	26	430
Hot mustard sauce	1 package	3	60
BBQ sauce	1 package	0	45
Sweet 'n sour sauce	1 package	0	50
Honey	1 package	0	45
Honey mustard	1 package	4	50
Sides & Salads			
French fries			
small	1 serving	10	210
large	1 serving	22	450
super-sized	1 serving	26	540
Fajita chicken salad	1 serving	6	160
Garden salad	1 serving	4	80
Blue cheese dressing	1 package	17	190
Ranch dressing	1 package	21	230
1000 island dressing	1 package	13	190
Lite vinaigrette	1 package	2	50
Red French reduced calorie	1 package	8	160
Desserts			
Vanilla low fat frozen yogurt cone	1 serving	1	120
Strby. low fat frzn. yogurt sundae	1 serving	1	240
Caramel low fat yogurt sundae	1 serving	3	310
Hot fudge sundae	1 serving	5	290
Nuts on sundaes	1 serving	3	40
Baked apple pie	1 serving	13	260
McDonaldland® cookies	1 serving	9	260
Vanilla shake	1 small	5	340
Chocolate shake	1 small	5	340
Strawberry shake	1 small	5	340

1 Potato 2®

Food Item	Amount	Fat Gm.	Calories
Potato Entrees			
Bacon & cheese	1 w/o skin	50	720
Bacon double cheeseburger	1 w/o skin	56	825
Broccoli & cheese	1 w/o skin	41	630
Butter potato	1 w/o skin	18	345

Food Item	Amount	Fat Gm.	Calories
1 Potato 2 (continued)			
Chicken, broccoli, & cheese	1 w/o skin	47	755
Chicken & broccoli lite	1 w/o skin	8	340
Chicken stir-fry lite	1 w/o skin	3	355
Crab, broccoli & cheese	1 w/o skin	37	660
Crab & broccoli DeLite	1 w/o skin	6	345
Ham and cheese	1 w/o skin	44	680
Ham, broccoli & ranch	1 w/o skin	66	950
Margarine potato	1 w/o skin	22	375
Mexican	1 w/o skin	44	665
Philly steak & cheese	1 w/o skin	51	850
Smoked turkey dijon lite	1 w/o skin	6	300
Sour cream & bacon	1 w/o skin	40	575
Sour cream & chives	1 w/o skin	30	460
SW grilled chicken lite	1 w/o skin	3	295
Spinach souffle lite	1 w/o skin	8	300
Steak teriyaki	1 w/o skin	38	645
Three cheese	1 w/o skin	44	670
Veggie & herb cheese, light	1 w/o skin	22	255
Potato Skins & Fries			
BBQ Chicken skins	1 serving	25	835
Bacon, cheddar & sour cream sn.	1 serving	59	1100
Mexiskins	1 serving	44	950
French fries			
8 oz..	1 serving	38	590
10 oz.	1 serving	47	740
16 oz.	1 serving	75	1185
Combos			
BBQ chicken & cheddar	1 serving	49	1010
Steak, mushroom & gravy	1 serving	47	955
Ham, peppers, onion & cheese	1 serving	51	965

Pizza Hut®

Food Item	Amount	Fat Gm.	Calories
Cheese			
Thin 'N Crispy®	1 slice med.	8	205
hand tossed	1 slice med.	7	235
pan	1 slice med.	11	260
Beef			
Thin 'N Crispy®	1 slice med.	11	225
hand tossed	1 slice med.	9	260
pan	1 slice med.	13	285
Ham			
Thin 'N Crispy®	1 slice med.	7	180
hand tossed	1 slice med.	5	210
pan	1 slice med.	9	235
Pepperoni			
Thin 'N Crispy®	1 slice med.	10	215
hand tossed	1 slice med.	8	235
pan	1 slice med.	12	265
Italian Sausage			
Thin 'N Crispy®	1 slice med.	12	235
hand tossed	1 slice med.	11	265
pan	1 slice med.	15	290
Pork Topping			
Thin 'N Crispy®	1 slice med.	12	235
hand tossed	1 slice med.	10	265
pan	1 slice med.	14	290
Meat Lover's®			
Thin 'N Crispy®	1 slice med.	13	285

Fast Food Nutritional Information

Food Item	Amount	Fat Gm.	Calories
Pizza Hut® (continued)			
hand tossed	1 slice med.	11	310
pan	1 slice med.	18	340
Veggie Lover's			
Thin 'N Crispy®	1 slice med.	7	185
hand tossed	1 slice med.	6	215
pan	1 slice med.	10	240
Pepperoni Lover's®			
Thin 'N Crispy®	1 slice med.	16	285
hand tossed	1 slice med.	14	305
pan	1 slice med.	17	330
Supreme			
Thin 'N Crispy®	1 slice med.	13	255
hand tossed	1 slice med.	12	280
pan	1 slice med.	15	310
Super Supreme			
Thin 'N Crispy®	1 slice med.	14	270
hand tossed	1 slice med.	13	295
pan	1 slice med.	17	320
Cheese Bigfoot™	1 slice BF	6	185
Pepperoni Bigfoot™	1 slice BF	7	205
Pep., mshrm, & Itl. sg. Bigfoot™	1 slice BF	8	210
Personal Pan Pizza®			
pepperoni	whole pizza	28	635
supreme	whole pizza	34	720

Taco Bell®

Tacos

Food Item	Amount	Fat Gm.	Calories
Taco	1 serving	11	180
Taco Supreme™	1 serving	15	230
Soft taco	1 serving	11	220
Soft Taco Supreme®	1 serving	15	270
Light chicken soft taco	1 serving	5	180
Double decker taco	1 serving	15	330
Double Decker Taco Supreme™	1 serving	18	370
Soft taco roll-up	1 serving	10	200

Burritos

Food Item	Amount	Fat Gm.	Calories
Bean burrito	1 serving	11	370
Burrito Supreme®	1 serving	18	430
Light chicken burrito	1 serving	6	290
Light chicken burrito Supreme®	1 serving	10	410
7-layer burrito	1 serving	21	510
Big Beef Burrito Supreme®	1 serving	24	510
Chili Cheese Burrito	1 serving	18	380

Extras

Food Item	Amount	Fat Gm.	Calories
Taco salad	1 serving	52	850
Pintos'n cheese	1 serving	7	170
Tostada	1 serving	10	230
Mexican pizza	1 serving	37	580
Beef MexiMelt®	1 serving	14	260
Nachos	1 serving	18	340
Nachos Supreme	1 serving	21	400
Nachos BellGrande®	1 serving	32	610
Cinnamon Twists	1 serving	6	140
Seasoned rice	1 serving	3	110

Sauces

Food Item	Amount	Fat Gm.	Calories
Green sauce	1 serving	0	5
Guacamole	1 serving	3	35

Food Item	Amount	Fat Gm.	Calories
Taco Bell® (continued)			
Taco sauce	1 serving	0	0
Nacho cheese sauce	1 serving	3	40
Picante sauce	1 serving	0	0
Pico de gallo	1 serving	0	5
Ranch dressing	1 serving	9	90
Red sauce	1 serving	0	10
Salsa	1 serving	0	30
Sour cream	1 serving	4	40
Non-fat sour cream	1 serving	0	15

Wendy's®

Sandwiches

Food Item	Amount	Fat Gm.	Calories
Plain single	1 serving	16	360
Single with everything	1 serving	20	420
Big bacon classic	1 serving	33	610
Jr. hamburger	1 serving	10	270
Jr. cheeseburger	1 serving	13	320
Jr. bacon cheeseburger	1 serving	21	410
Jr. cheeseburger deluxe	1 serving	16	360
Hamburger, kids' meal	1 serving	10	270
Cheeseburger, kids' meal	1 serving	13	320
Grilled chicken sandwich	1 serving	7	290
Breaded chicken sandwich	1 serving	18	440
Chicken club sandwich	1 serving	23	500

Food Item	Amount	Fat Gm.	Calories
French Fries			
small	1 serving	13	260
medium	1 serving	19	380
biggie	1 serving	23	460
Baked potato			
plain	1 serving	0	310
bacon & cheese	1 serving	18	540
broccoli & cheese	1 serving	14	470
cheese	1 serving	23	570
chili & cheese	1 serving	24	620
sour cream & chives	1 serving	6	380
Chili			
small	8 oz.	7	210
large	12 oz.	10	310
cheddar cheese, shredded	2 T.	6	70
Chicken nuggets	6 pieces	20	280
Barbeque sauce	1 packet	0	50
Honey	1 packet	0	45
Sweet & sour sauce	1 packet	0	45
Sweet mustard sauce	1 packet	1	50

Salads-To-Go

Food Item	Amount	Fat Gm.	Calories
Caesar side salad	1 salad	5	110
Deluxe garden salad	1 salad	6	110
Grilled chicken salad	1 salad	8	200
Side salad	1 salad	3	60
Taco salad	1 salad	30	590
Soft breadstick	1 stick	3	130

Desserts

Food Item	Amount	Fat Gm.	Calories
Chocolate chip cookie	1 each	11	270
Frosty™ dairy dessert			
small	1 serving	10	340
medium	1 serving	13	460
large	1 serving	17	570

Fast Food Tips

In today's busy world, fast foods are a great convenience. By checking the food values before ordering, you can have a satisfying meal with a reasonable amount of fat and calories. For breakfasts, try English muffins with jelly or pancakes with syrup. Avoid egg dishes and breakfast sandwiches. Here are some sample lunch and dinner menus that show you how to build your own meal.

	Amt.	Fat g.	Cal.
Burger King®			
Chunky Chicken Salad	1	4	142
Italian dressing, lo-cal	2 T.	2	30
Diet cola	1 med.	0	1
Totals		6	173
Chicken Tenders	6 piece	13	236
Baked potato	1 med.	0	210
Coffee	1	0	2
Totals		13	448
Hardees®			
Regular roast beef	1	11	270
Side salad	1	0	20
Low-cal dressing	1	1	30
Water	1	0	0
Totals		12	320
McDonald's®			
McGrilled Chic. Sand.	1	4	260
Side Salad	1	1	30
'Lite' vinaigrette	1/2 pg.	1	24
1% milk	8 oz.	2	110
Totals		8	424
Chicken fajita	1	8	190
Vanilla yogurt cone	1	1	105
Orange juice	1	0	80
Totals		9	375

	Amt.	Fat g.	Cal.
Pizza Hut®			
Chunky Veggie, hnd. tsd.	2 sl.	12	448
Diet cola	1	0	0
Totals		12	448
Subway®			
6" turkey breast sub	1	10	320
Diet Pepsi	1	0	0
Totals		10	320
Small roast beef salad	1	10	220
2% milk	1	5	120
Totals		15	340
Taco Bell®			
Chicken Soft Taco	1	10	213
Diet cola	1	0	0
Totals		10	213
Wendy's®			
Chili	sm.	6	190
Plain baked potato	1	0	310
Iced tea	1	0	0
Totals	1	6	500
Chicken Sandwich	1	7	290
Side salad	1	3	60
Fat-free dressing	2 T.	0	35
Diet cola	1	0	0
Totals		10	385

How to Make Better Choices When Eating Out

• Shop carefully for a restaurant that is more likely to accommodate special requests. A telephone call ahead of time can be helpful when choosing a restaurant.

• Don't skip a meal on a day you're going out to eat. In fact, have a light snack an hour or so before leaving home to avoid over-eating at the restaurant.

• Food in the diet or light section of the menu often has far more calories and fat than you might suspect. Look for meals that contain little or no fat, small amounts of meat, poultry, or fish, lots of vegetables and a low fat source of carbohydrates such as a baked potato, rice, or bread.

• Ordering "a' la carte" can cost more, but it allows you to eat what you want. Look for appetizers that are broiled, baked, or steamed—not deep-fried in fat.

• Ask your server to clarify unfamiliar terms or to explain how a dish is prepared. Request smaller portions and ask that dressings and sauces be served on the side. Request modified cooking methods (broiling instead of frying, for example).

• Etiquette and nutrition often go hand-in-hand. Don't gulp your food. Chew thoroughly. Eating slowly helps digestion and keeps you from stuffing yourself (it takes 20 minutes before the brain realizes the stomach is full). Practice techniques to extend mealtimes without eating more food: put down your fork between bites, focus on the conversation, or share your meal with a companion. This limits your caloric intake and gives you two meals for the price of one.

• For dessert, share with a friend or take half home. Request sherbet, angel food cake, low fat yogurt or just an after-dinner mint if you want something sweet at the end of your meal.

• If you choose the salad bar, be careful what you pile on your plate (especially toppings and salad dressing). Survey the entire bar before deciding what's best for you. Start with plenty of lettuce, veggies, and low fat dressing. *Then* add the other goodies; that way you'll be more likely to take less of them. Don't forget that a salad piled high with toppings and dressing can be higher in fat and calories than a meat and potatoes meal! The nutritional low-down on most salad bar favorites is listed below.

Common Salad Bar Ingredients:

	Amt.	Fat g.	Cal.		Amt.	Fat g.	Cal.
Avocado	1/4	8	81	Parmesan cheese	1 T.	2	23
Bacon Bits	1 T.	2	40	Radishes	1 T.	0	2
Broccoli	1/4 C.	0	6	Salad greens	1 C.	0	10
Carrots	1 T.	0	1	Sunflower seeds	1 T.	5	52
Cauliflower	1/4 C.	0	6	Tomato	2 sl.	0	5
Cheddar cheese	1 T.	2	29	Turkey chunks	1/4 C.	2	70
Cottage cheese 2%	1/2 C.	2	102				
Cucumbers	1 T.	0	2	**Dressing**			
Garbanzo beans	1 T.	0	17	Blue cheese	2 T.	19	180
Green pepper	1 T.	0	2	French	2 T.	11	120
Ham chunks	1/4 C.	8	120	Italian	2 T.	14	140
Hard cooked eggs	1/2	3	39	Italian, low-cal.	2 T.	3	40
Mushrooms	1 T.	0	0	Ranch	2 T.	15	180
Olives	5 lg.	2	26	Ranch, low-cal.	2 T.	9	120
Onions	1 T.	0	2	Thousand Island	2 T.	13	130

The Food Label

What Does it *Really* Mean?

Most foods in the grocery store must now have a nutritional label. Look at the "Nutrition Facts" on a product label for specific information on serving size and nutrients, including total fat, cholesterol and sodium.

Nutrient claims like "low fat" can only be used if a food meets legal standards as defined by the U.S. government.

Fat-free   Less than 0.5 grams of
                      fat per serving

Low Fat   3 fat grams or less
                      per serving

Reduced Fat   At least 25% less fat per serving compared to similar food

Cholesterol-free Less than 2 mg. cholesterol and 2 grams or less saturated fat per serving

Low Cholesterol   20 mg. or less cholesterol and 2 grams or less saturated fat per serving

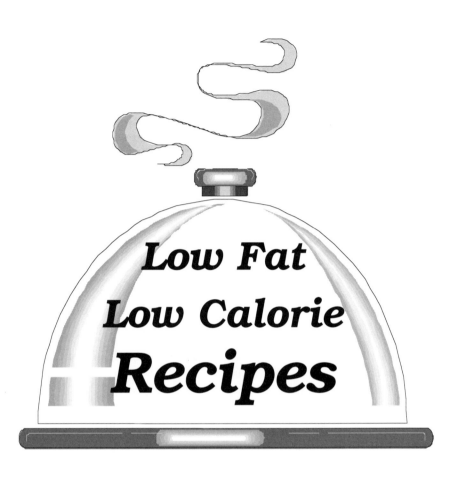

Low Fat
Low Calorie
Recipes

Bon appétit!

Chicken Spread

Makes 1 cup—15 calories & 1 fat gram per tablespoon

1 cup chicken finely chopped
1 T. crushed pineapple, drained
1/8 tsp. salt

1 T. chopped celery
1/4 tsp. curry powder
1 T. mayo-type dressing

Mix together well. Spread on unsalted whole-grain crackers or in mini pita pockets. Keeps in refrigerator for 3-4 days.

Ham & Cheese Roll-Ups

Serves 4—71 calories & 5 fat grams per serving

2 oz. Neufchatel cheese, softened
2 tsp. low-cal. mayonnaise
1/3 cup alfalfa sprouts

4 slices lean ham
3/4 tsp. prepared mustard

Combine Neufchatel cheese, mayo, and mustard. Spread evenly over ham slices and top with sprouts. Roll up, jelly roll style. Secure with toothpicks in 1-inch increments. Chill. Before serving, slice between toothpicks.

Honey Mustard Chicken Chunks

Serves 6—126 calories & 3 fat grams per 3 chunks

1/4 cup honey
2 T. prepared mustard
1 T. low cal. margarine
2 skinless, boneless chicken breasts, cut into 18 1" chunks

1/2 cup cornflake crumbs
1 tsp. paprika
2 tsp. soy sauce

Microwave honey, mustard, margarine and soy sauce on high for 20 seconds. Divide sauce. Add chicken to one half of the sauce and stir to coat evenly. Combine cornflake crumbs and paprika. Dredge chicken through dry ingredients and discard remaining sauce. Microwave chicken on high for 2 minutes, 9 pieces at a time. Microwave remaining half of sauce on high for 1-1 1/2 minutes. Serve chicken chunks and sauce with a toothpick in each chunk.

Layered Mexican Dip
35 calories & 0 fat grams per serving

8 oz. fat-free cream cheese
8 oz. fat-free sour cream
1 pkg. taco seasoning mix
1 cup chopped lettuce

2 chopped tomatoes
2 gr. onions, chopped finely
8 oz. grated fat-free
   cheddar cheese

Blend together cream cheese, sour cream and taco seasoning mix. Spread on a platter. Top with chopped lettuce, tomatoes, green onions and grated cheese. Serve with low-fat taco chips or baked tortillas. Salsa can also be drizzled over top if desired.

Mexican Snack Pizzas
95 calories & 2 fat grams per 1/2 muffin

2 whole-wheat English muffins
1/4 cup kidney beans, drained and chopped
1 T. green pepper, chopped
1/4 cup mozzarella cheese, grated

1/4 cup tomato pureé
1 T. chopped onion
1/2 tsp. oregano leaves
1/4 cup shredded lettuce

Split muffins and toast. Mix pureé, beans, onion, green pepper, and oregano. Spread on muffin halves. Sprinkle with cheese. Broil until cheese melts. Garnish with lettuce.

Pineapple Cheese Spread
Makes 1 cup—35 calories & 2 fat grams per tablespoon

6 oz. mozzarella cheese,
   part skim milk
1 T. pineapple juice

1/3 cup crushed pineapple,
   canned & drained

Cut cheese into small pieces. Mix ingredients in blender or food processor, scraping sides often. When mixture is smooth and creamy, serve on unsalted whole-wheat crackers.

Breads

Cheesey Sausage Biscuits
Makes 1 dozen biscuits—68 calories & 2 fat grams

1/4 pound raw turkey sausage
1/2 cup all-purpose flour
1/2 cup unprocessed oat bran
1/2 cup (2 oz.) low cal. grated cheddar cheese

1 tsp. baking powder
1/8 tsp. baking soda
1/2 cup + 3 T. buttermilk
cooking oil spray

Brown sausage, drain. Combine with remaining dry ingredients; add buttermilk, stirring until moistened. Bake spoonfuls of dough on sprayed baking sheet at 450° 11 minutes.

Herb Corn Bread
Makes 2 loaves—80 calories & 3 fat grams per 1/2" slice

1 cup all-purpose flour
1 cup yellow cornmeal
2 T. sugar
2 tsp. baking powder
2 tsp. fresh, minced thyme
2 tsp. fresh, minced chives
1 1/2 tsp. grated lemon rind
1/8 tsp. salt

1/8 tsp. pepper
1/2 cup corn cut from cob
1 cup non-fat yogurt
3 T. vegetable oil
1 T. water
1 egg, beaten
cooking oil spray

Combine first 10 ingredients. Mix yogurt, oil, water and egg. Stir into flour mixture until moist. Spoon into two lightly sprayed loaf pans. Bake at 400° for 25 minutes.

Oatmeal Muffins
Makes 15 muffins—100 calories & 2 fat grams

1/2 cup shreds of wheat bran cereal
1 cup buttermilk
1 cup finely grated carrot
1 T. vegetable oil
2 eggs, beaten
1 cup quick-cooking oats, uncooked

3/4 cup all-purpose flour
1/2 cup packed brown sugar
1 tsp. baking powder
1/2 tsp. baking soda
2 tsp. ground cinnamon
1/4 tsp. salt

Soak cereal in milk for 2 minutes. Add carrot, oil, and eggs, stir. Combine dry ingredients and add to mixture, stirring until moist. Place in double cupcake liners and microwave 6 at a time on high for 2-2 1/2 minutes.

Breads

Pumpkin & Oatmeal Bread
Makes 2 loaves—157 calories & 7 fat grams per 1/2" slice

3 cups sifted all-purpose flour
1 cup oats
1 T. + 1 tsp. baking powder
2 tsp. cinnamon
1 tsp. baking soda
1 tsp. salt
1 tsp. ginger
1 tsp. mace
1/4 tsp. ground cloves

1 cup honey
1/2 cup vegetable oil
4 eggs, lightly beaten
2/3 cup orange juice
1 16 oz. can pumpkin
1 cup chopped pecans
cooking oil spray
1 egg white, lightly beaten
1/4 cup oats

Combine dry ingredients. Mix honey, oil, and eggs; add to flour mixture. Add juice, pumpkin, and pecans. Top loaf w/ egg white and oats; bake 350° 1 hr. in 2 sprayed loaf pans.

Strawberry Scones
Makes 1 dozen—147 calories & 4 fat grams per scone

2 cups flour
1 8-oz. carton vanilla low fat yogurt
1/4 cup non-sweetened strawberry or raspberry spread
1/2 tsp. baking soda
3 T. margarine, chilled and cut into small pieces

cooking oil spray
1/4 cup sugar
2 tsp. baking powder
1/4 tsp. salt
2 T. finely chopped pecans

Combine dry ingredients, cut in margarine with pastry blender. Stir in yogurt. Knead dough on floured board; pat into 8" circle on sprayed baking sheet. Cut into 12 wedges. Slit each wedge and fill with fruit spread; top w/ pecans. Bake 13 minutes at 400°.

Cinnamon Biscuits
Makes 1 dozen—153 calories & 3 fat grams per biscuit

2 cups all-purpose flour
2 tsp. baking powder
1 1/2 T. sugar
1/2 tsp. cinnamon
1/4 tsp. salt

3 T. chilled stick margarine
1/2 cup raisins
3/4 cup 1% milk
1/2 cup powdered sugar
1 T. 1% milk

Mix dry ingredients, cut in margarine. Add raisins & milk; mix. Knead, cut out biscuits. Bake 11 minutes at 450°. Mix powdered sugar and 1 T. milk. Spread over biscuits.

Soups & Salads

Beef-Potato Soup
Makes 5 cups—120 calories & 3 fat grams per 1 1/4 cup serving

1/3 pound ground beef, drained
1 cup sliced onions
salt & pepper to taste
1 bay leaf
1 1/2 cups sliced potatoes

3 cups water
1/2 cup chopped celery
2 tsp. chopped parsley
2 whole cloves
1/2 cup grated carrots

Brown beef; drain fat. Add water, onions, celery, and seasonings. Boil; reduce heat and cook for 30 minutes. Add potatoes, carrots, and parsley. Cook until potatoes are tender, about 15 minutes. Remove bay leaf and cloves before serving.

Luncheon Chicken Salad
Makes 6 1-cup servings—183 calories & 4 fat grams

2 cups cubed, cooked chicken breast
1 cup cubed, unpeeled Red Delicious apple
2/3 cup celery, sliced diagonally
1/3 cup plain non-fat yogurt
1 1/2 T. lemon juice
1 T. chopped fresh celery leaves

1 1/2 C. seedless red grapes
1/4 cup raisins
2 T. diced purple onion
2 T. low-cal. mayonnaise
1/4 tsp. salt
6 Boston lettuce leaves

Combine chicken, apple, celery, grapes, raisins, and onion in bowl. Blend remaining ingredients and toss with salad. Chill. Serve on individual lettuce-lined serving plates.

Chicken Stew
Makes 4 1-cup servings—175 calories & 2 fat grams

2 chicken breast halves w/o skin
2/3 cup frozen mixed vegetables
2/3 cup diced potatoes
1/4 tsp. ground thyme
1/4 cup flour

1/2 cup chopped onion
1/4 cup sliced celery
1 cup chopped tomatoes
1/8 tsp. pepper
1/4 cup water

Cook chicken in water with salt, 2 cloves, and 1 bay leaf for 45 minutes until tender. Cut up meat. Discard leaf and cloves, add water to make 2 cups. Cook veggies in broth for 10 minutes. Add tomatoes and spices. Simmer for 15 minutes. Add chicken. Mix flour and water until smooth. Add to stew, stirring until thickened.

Soups & Salads

Chicken Chutney Salad
Serves 6—259 calories & 5 fat grams per serving

6 cups loosely packed sliced romaine leaves
2 T. chopped almonds
1 1/2 pounds skinned, boned chicken breast
1 9-oz. jar mango chutney

1/2 cup sliced green onions
vegetable cooking spray
1 cup celery, slice diagonally

Toast almonds for 8 minutes in 350° oven; set aside. Spray skillet with oil and cook chicken until done, about 7 minutes per side. Cut across grain into thin slices. Toss chicken, almonds, chutney, onions, and celery all together until well coated. Spoon onto 6 individual lettuce-lined plates.

Vegetable Soup
Makes 4 1-cup servings—70 calories & 0 fat grams

1 cup diced potatoes
1/2 cup chopped onion
1/2 cup sliced carrots
1/4 tsp. oregano leaves
salt and pepper to taste
1 cup tomatoes

1 cup chopped cabbage
1/2 cup diced celery
1/2 cup frozen green beans
1/4 tsp. marjoram leaves
1 bay leaf
2 cups water

Place all ingredients except tomatoes in saucepan and simmer about 10 minutes. Add tomatoes and cook an additional 20 minutes. Discard bay leaf before serving.

Pear & Snow Pea Salad
Serves 4—95 calories & 3 fat grams

1/4 cup plain non-fat yogurt
2 T. unsweetened pineapple juice
3 green onions, thinly sliced
1/2 pound fresh snow peas, trimmed
2 T. chopped, toasted walnuts

1 tsp. lime juice
8 radicchio leaves
1/2 tsp. sugar
1 large firm, ripe pear

Combine yogurt, sugar, and pineapple juice; set aside. Boil snow peas for 15 seconds; cool and pat dry. Cut pear in half lengthwise; core and cut lengthwise again into thin slices. Brush cut sides with lime juice. Arrange snow peas and pears on radicchio-lined salad plates. Drizzle yogurt mixture over top and sprinkle with green onions and walnuts.

Entrees

Tropical Swordfish
Makes 4 servings—178 calories & 5 fat grams

1/2 cup chopped ripe mango
2 T. finely chopped celery
2 tsp. finely chopped purple onion
1 tsp. seeded, minced jalapeno pepper
2 T. rice vinegar
1 T. + 1 tsp. low sodium soy sauce

1/4 C. peeled, chopped papaya
1 T. minced fresh parsley
1 T. lime juice
1 tsp. grated, fresh ginger
2 T. Dijon mustard
4 swordfish steaks

Combine rice vinegar, mustard and soy sauce. Brush over swordfish steaks. Spray grill with cooking oil and grill steaks about 5 minutes per side, or until it flakes easily. While fish cooks, combine remaining ingredients. Serve fish with 1/4 cup mango mixture. Garnish with parsley sprig.

Beef-Vegetable Stir-Fry
Makes 4 3/4-cup servings—180 calories & 6 fat grams

12 oz. beef round steak, boneless
1/2 cup sliced carrots
1/2 cup sliced onions
1/8 tsp. garlic powder
2 cups zucchini, cut into thin strips

1 tsp. oil
1/2 cup sliced celery
1 T. soy sauce
1 dash pepper
2 T. stir-fry sauce or glaze

Brown meat in oil until no longer red. Reduce heat. Add carrots, celery, onion, and seasonings. Cover and cook until carrots are slightly tender, 3-4 minutes. Add squash, cook until vegetables are tender-crisp, 3 to 4 minutes. Add stir-fry glaze. Stir until all is lightly coated with glaze.

Enchilada Casserole
Serves 4—300 calories & 5 fat grams

1/2 cup chopped onion
1/2 cup chopped green pepper
1/2 cup canned, drained pinto beans
3/4 cup water
1/8 tsp. ground cumin
1/2 cup tomato pureé
1 1/2 cup tomato pureé

1/4 cup chopped celery
1 cup diced, cooked chicken
1/8 tsp. salt
1 T. chili powder
1/8 tsp. garlic powder
1/4 C gr. Monterey Jack cheese
whole wheat tortillas

Preheat oven to 350°. Simmer onion, green pepper, and celery until tender, drain. Add chicken, beans, and 1/2 the pureé; mix. In baking pan place 4 tortillas, half the filling mixture, and 1/4 of the sauce. Add remaining filling and 1/4 of sauce. Cover with 4 tortillas and remaining sauce. Sprinkle cheese over top. Bake until cheese is melted and sauce bubbly, about 30 minutes.

Entrees

Pork-Sweet Potato Skillet
Serves 4—270 calories and 6 fat grams

4 thin-cut pork chops
1 cup apple juice
1 medium onion, sliced
1 T. flour

1/8 tsp. ground allspice
1/8 tsp. salt
1 17 oz. can sweet potatoes

Brown chops on both sides. Add 3/4 cup apple juice. Top with onion slices. Cover and cook 5 minutes, reduce heat. Mix flour and seasonings. Stir into remaining 1/4 cup apple juice. Stir into pan. Place sweet potatoes in pan, spooning sauce over. Cover and cook an additional 10 minutes, or until chops are done.

Pork & Pepper Stir-Fry
Serves 4—166 calories & 4 fat grams

1 pound pork tenderloin
1 T. low-sodium soy sauce
1/4 tsp. ground ginger
1 cup slivered onion
3/4 cup red pepper, julienne cut
3/4 cup yellow pepper, julienne cut

1 tsp. dark sesame oil
1/4 tsp. garlic powder
1/4 tsp. ground cumin
3/4 cup gr. pepper, julienne
2 T. white wine vinegar

Trim fat from pork and cut cross-wise in 1/4" slices. Stir-fry pork, soy sauce, garlic powder, ginger, and cumin about 3 minutes. Remove pork and set aside. Stir-fry onion and peppers about 5 minutes. Return pork, add vinegar and cook an additional minute.

Pizza
Serves 4—275 calories & 6 fat grams

1 can refrigerated pizza crust
3/4 cup canned tomato pureé (no salt)
1 small onion, sliced
1 cup fresh mushrooms, sliced

1 tsp. oregano leaves
1/2 tsp. garlic powder
1/2 sm. green pepper, sliced
1 cup shredded mozzarella

Preheat oven to 450°. Spread dough on ungreased cookie sheet. Mix pureé and seasonings together, spread evenly over crust. Top with vegetables and sprinkle with cheese. Bake until cheese melts, about 15 minutes.

Entrees

Low Fat Fried Chicken
Serves 8—220 calories & 11 fat grams

1 3-pound chicken (skinned with bones)
2 egg whites whisked with 2 T. lemon juice
1/2 cup dry whole wheat bread crumbs
1/4 cup parmesan cheese

1 tsp. dry parsley
1/2 tsp. paprika
1 tsp. rosemary

Remove skin from chicken, rinse and pat dry. Dip chicken pieces in egg white/lemon mixture, then dredge in dry mixture. Spray foil-lined jelly roll pan with non-stick coating. Bake in 400° oven for 40-45 minutes.

Orange-Mustard Glazed Turkey Cutlets
Serves 4—160 calories & 3 fat grams

2 T. frozen orange juice concentrate
1 tsp. stone-ground mustard
8 turkey cutlets

4 cloves garlic, crushed
vegetable oil spray
2 tsp. low calorie margarine

Combine orange juice with mustard; set aside. Pierce both sides of cutlets with a fork and rub with garlic on both sides. Spray skillet with oil, add margarine and cook cutlets about 2 minutes per side. Turn down heat to low. Add orange juice mixture and stir, thoroughly coating cutlets.

Quick Chili
Serves 4—220 calories & 8 fat grams

1/2 pound lean ground beef (rinsed)
1 16-oz. can kidney beans, drained (save liquid)
1/3 cup bean liquid

1 T. instant minced onion
1 1/2 tsp. chili powder
1 C. tomato pureé, unsalted

Cook beef and drain fat. Add remaining ingredients. Bring to a boil, reduce heat, cover and simmer at least 10 minutes.

Entrees

Individual Meat Loaves
Makes 4 individual loaves—200 calories & 11 fat grams

3/4 pound extra-lean ground beef
1/3 cup crushed wheat crackers
1/2 tsp. basil leaves
1 T. instant minced onion

1 egg
1/3 cup skim milk
1/8 tsp. salt

Preheat oven to 375°. Soak crackers and onion in milk; add egg and seasonings. Mix well. Add ground beef; mix and form into four loaves. Bake in shallow baking pan about 25 minutes or until done. Drain off fat.

Microwaved Stuffed Peppers
Serves 4—215 calories & 12 fat grams

2 green peppers, halved and seeded
boiling water to cover peppers

1/4 cup tomato sauce
meat loaf mixture (above)

Cook peppers in boiling water for 2 minutes. Drain well. Fill pepper halves with meat mixture and place in glass baking dish. Spread 1 T. tomato sauce over each serving. Cover with wax paper. Microwave on high power for 7 minutes. Rotate dish halfway through cooking. Remove from oven and let stand, covered, about 3 minutes.

Aloha Meatballs
Serves 4—245 calories & 11 fat grams

1 recipe meat loaf mixture (top recipe)
1 8 oz. can pineapple chunks, juice packed
1 1/2 tsp. Worcestershire sauce
1/2 cup green pepper, cut into 1" pieces

1 dash pepper
1 T. cornstarch
1 T. water
1/4 tsp. garlic powder

Shape meat mixture into 12 balls. Brown meatballs, about 10 minutes; drain. Drain pineapple, saving juice. Add enough water to juice to make 3/4 cup liquid. Add liquid and seasonings to pan. Boil, reduce heat, cover, and cook an additional 5 minutes. Add pineapple chunks and green pepper. Cook 1 minute. Stir cornstarch and water together; add to pan and stir until thickened.

Side Dishes

Stuffed Baked Potato
Serves 4—155 calories & 0 fat grams

4 baking potatoes
1/2 cup fat-free cottage cheese
1/8 tsp. pepper

3 T. skim milk
1 tsp. dried chopped chives
paprika

Wash and pierce potatoes; bake at 425° for 1 hour. Cut off tops of potatoes lengthwise. Scoop out potatoes, mix with blended cottage cheese, milk, and seasonings. Stuff potato skins, sprinkle with paprika and bake an additional 10 minutes.

Rice-Pasta Pilaf
Serves 4—135 calories & 4 fat grams

1/3 cup uncooked brown rice
1 1/2 cup unsalted chicken broth
2 tsp. margarine
2 T. chopped green onions
2 T. chopped green pepper
2 oz. thin spaghetti, broken into 1/2"-1" pieces

2 T. chopped mushrooms
1/2 clove minced garlic
1/2 tsp. savory
1/8 tsp. pepper
1/4 tsp. salt
1/3 cup slivered almonds

Cook rice in 1 cup broth, about 35 minutes. Brown spaghetti in margarine 2 minutes. Add 1/2 cup broth, vegetables, & rice. Boil. Cover and reduce heat. Cook until moisture is absorbed, about 10 minutes. Garnish with toasted almonds.

Lemon & Herb Veggies
Serves 4—50 calories & 2 fat grams

1 16-oz. pkg. frozen broccoli, carrots, & cauliflower
3 T. cooking water
1 1/2 tsp. dry basil or 1/4 cup fresh
1/4 tsp. cracked black pepper

2 T. lemon juice
1 clove garlic, minced
1 1/2 tsp. margarine
1/2 tsp. chic. bouillon grains

Cook vegetables in 1/4 cup water, covered until done; drain but reserve liquid. Dissolve bouillon in 3 T. cooking water. Melt margarine in microwave dish, add garlic and cook on high for 30 seconds. Stir in broth, lemon juice, and seasoning. Cook for 2 minutes until thickened. Gently stir into hot vegetables.

Side Dishes

Mini Sweet Potato Casseroles
Serves 4—188 calories & 1 fat gram

4 cup peeled, cubed sweet potato
1/4 cup unsweetened apple juice
1 1/2 T. brown sugar
2 T. buttermilk
2 T. fat-free sour cream
1 tsp. grated orange rind
1 tsp. crushed Gingersnap cookie

1/8 tsp. ground cinnamon
1/8 tsp. ground coriander
1/8 tsp. ground nutmeg
2 egg whites
cooking oil spray
1 tsp. chopped pecans
1/4 tsp. orange extract

Pureé cooked sweet potato in food processor. Mix with apple juice, brown sugar, milk, sour cream, rind, extract, and spices. Let cool. Beat egg whites to stiff peaks, gently fold into potato mixture. Spoon into 4 individual, sprayed mini-casserole dishes. Sprinkle with crushed cookie and chopped pecans. Place casseroles in pan; pour hot water into pan to a depth of 1". Bake at 325° for 30 minutes.

Quick Five Bean Salad
Makes 10 servings—120 calories & 1 fat gram

1 16-oz. can green beans
1 16-oz. can kidney beans
1 16-oz. can garbanzo beans
1 chopped green pepper
1 1/4 cup sugar
dash black pepper

1 16-oz. can wax beans
1 16-oz. can lima beans
1/2 cup chopped onion
1 cup vinegar
2 tsp. oil

Drain all cans of beans. Mix ingredients all together in bowl and chill.

Baked Potato Wedges
Serves 4—122 calories & 0 fat grams

4 washed potatoes
cajun seasoning

cooking oil spray
garlic or seasoning salt

Slice each potato into 8 wedges and spray potatoes with non-fat cooking oil spray. Place on sprayed cookie sheet and sprinkle with seasoning. Bake at 450° for 15-20 minutes or until lightly browned. Serve with fat-free sour cream or salsa.

Desserts

Snow-Frosted Chocolate Brownies
Makes 1 1/2 dozen—97 calories & 4 fat grams per bar

1/2 cup low-calorie margarine
1/4 cup unsweetened cocoa
1 tsp. baking powder
1 1/2 tsp. vanilla extract, divided

1 tsp. chocolate extract
1 cup sugar, divided
3/4 cup flour
3 egg whites, divided

Melt margarine and cocoa. Mix in bowl with flour, baking powder, 3/4 cup sugar, 1 tsp. vanilla, extract, and 2 egg whites. Spread in 9" sprayed pan. Beat remaining egg white to stiff peaks. Slowly add remaining sugar & fold in remaining vanilla. Drop spoonfuls of egg whites evenly over mixture and swirl a knife through whites and batter in both directions. Bake at 325° for 25 minutes or until meringue is set and browned. Cool on rack.

Moist Mocha Cake
Serves 9—221 calories and 6 fat grams

1 cup flour
1 cup sugar, divided
1/4 cup + 2 T. unsweetened cocoa, divided
1 1/2 T. instant coffee granules
2 tsp. baking powder
1 cup + 2 T. vanilla ice milk

1/2 cup 1% milk
3 T. vegetable oil
1 tsp. vanilla extract
1 cup boiling water
1/4 tsp. salt
cooking oil spray

Combine flour, 2/3 cup sugar, 1/4 cup cocoa, coffee, baking powder, and salt; mix well. Mix milk, oil, and vanilla and add to dry ingredients; stir well. Spread into sprayed 8" pan. Mix 1/3 cup sugar + 2 T. cocoa. Sprinkle over batter. Pour 1 cup boiling water over batter (do not stir). Bake at 350° for 30 minutes. Serve warm, topped with ice milk.

Peanut Butter Cookies
Makes 4 dozen—48 calories & 2 fat grams per cookie

3/4 cup sugar
1/3 cup peanut butter
1/4 cup margarine, softened
2 egg whites

1 3/4 cup flour
1 tsp. baking soda
1/4 tsp. salt
1/2 tsp. vanilla extract

Combine first 3 ingredients w/ mixer. Add egg whites and vanilla; mix well. Add dry ingredients and mix well. Cover and chill 1 hr. Bake on sprayed sheet at 375° for 10 minutes.

Desserts

Individual Lime Souffles
Serves 6—100 calories & 3 fat grams

3 eggs, separated
1/3 cup sugar
1/4 cup fresh lime juice
2 T. flour
1 1/4 tsp. grated lime rind

2 egg whites
1/8 tsp. salt
1/8 tsp. cream of tartar
2 tsp. powdered sugar

Beat egg yolks with mixer, 5 minutes. Add 2 T. sugar, lime juice, flour, and rind. Set aside. Beat 5 egg whites until foamy. Add salt, cr. of tartar, and beat to soft peaks. Slowly add 3 T. + 1 tsp. sugar, beat to stiff peaks. Stir 1/4 egg white mixture into yolk mixture. Fold in remaining egg whites. Spoon into 6 sprayed individual soufflé cups. Bake at 350° for 10 minutes until puffed and golden. Sprinkle w/ powdered sugar. Serve hot.

Pumpkin Cupcakes
Makes 2 dozen—140 calories & 6 fat grams

1 1/2 cups whole wheat flour
1 cup all-purpose flour
3/4 cup sugar
2 T. baking powder
1/2 tsp. ground cinnamon
1/2 tsp. ground nutmeg
1/4 tsp. salt

3 eggs, slightly beaten
1 cup skim milk
1/2 cup oil
1 cup canned pumpkin
3/4 cup chopped raisins
1 T. vanilla

Mix dry ingreds. Mix remaining ingreds. and add to dry; mix. Bake 350° for 20 minutes.

Crunchy-Topped Chocolate Cake
Serves 8—195 calories & 6 fat grams

1/2 cup buttermilk
3 T. oil
1 egg
3/4 cup flour
1/2 cup wheat bran cereal flakes, crushed

3 T. unsweetened cocoa
1/2 tsp. baking soda
1/2 tsp. almond extract
2/3 cup packed brown sugar
2 T. brown sugar

Beat milk, oil, and egg for 1 minute; add extract. Mix flour, 2/3 cup brown sugar, baking soda, and cocoa. Stir into wet mixture; beat 2 minutes. Put in 8" pan, top w/ cereal and 2 T. brown sugar. Microwave on medium for 6 minutes, rotate after 1 minute.

A Final Word

You made it through 90 days! That's quite an achievement. By now you should be considerably more aware of calories and fat grams when making food selections. You're more conscious of what, and more importantly *why*, you were over-eating. This is the beginning of a lifetime of healthier eating.

If you have more weight to lose, continue recording your food choices and the emotions that influence them. Don't be discouraged if you're losing weight slowly; what's important is that you're consistently moving in the right direction. You now have the knowledge and determination to become thinner. Your new habits will slowly but surely find you realizing your ultimate goal.

Once you've achieved your desired weight, keep your journal close by so that you can review it should you find yourself slipping back into unhealthy patterns. Reviewing the emotions that plagued you in the past and seeing how you learned to overcome them will strengthen your resolve to get back on track.

Bradley Books is very proud to have assisted you on your journey toward improved fitness and health. We're glad to have provided you with useful information, encouragement, and some light-hearted thoughts along the way. Your comments or suggestions for this or other Bradley Books will be warmly received. Congratulations on an admirable achievement!

Notes: